METABOLIC CONFUSION MEAL PLAN FOR ENDOMORPH

Tailored Nutrition, Transformative Workouts, and a 28-day Meal Plan to Boost Your Metabolism, Ignite Weight Loss, and Enhance Overall Well-being

MICHELLE O. LEWIS

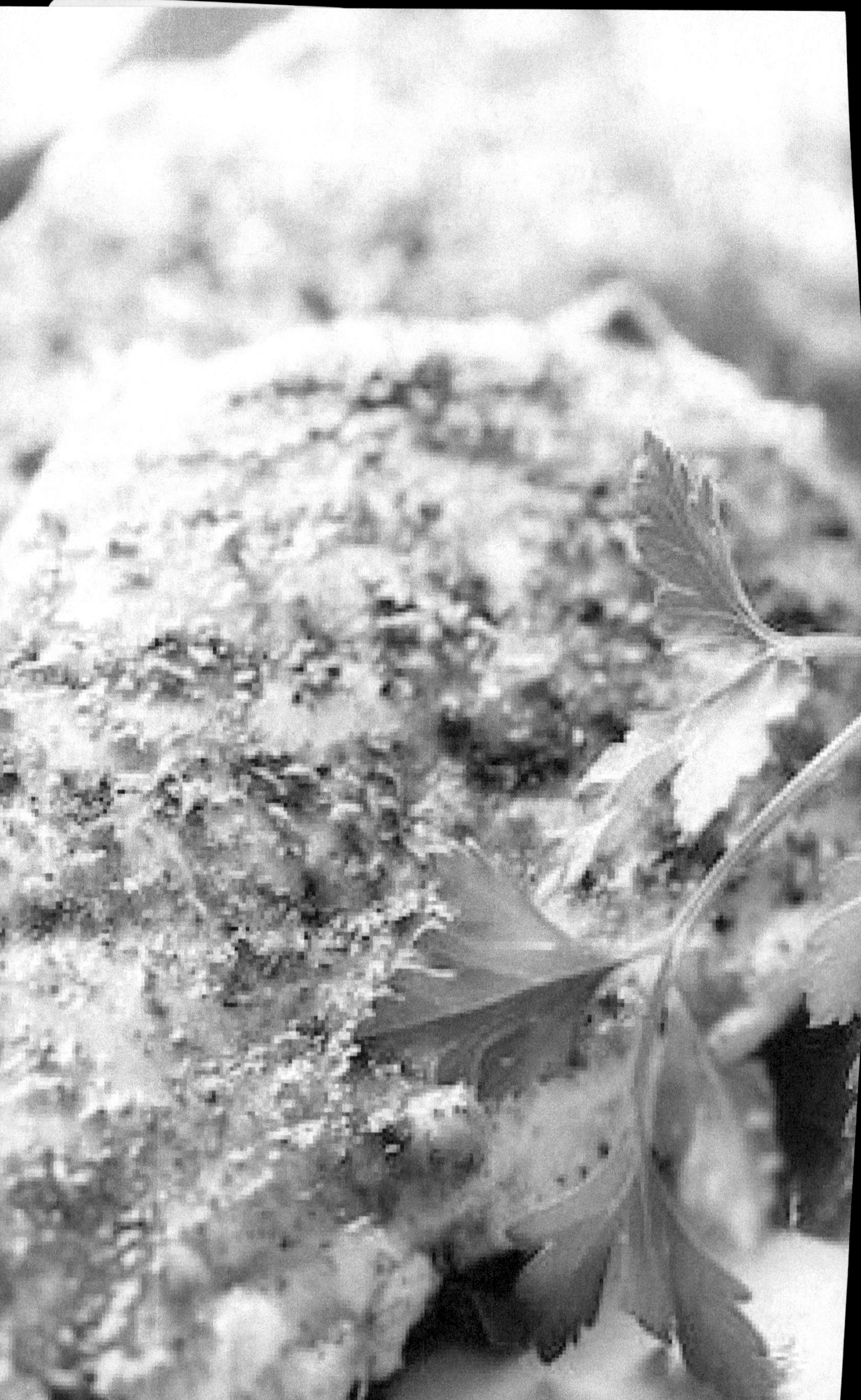

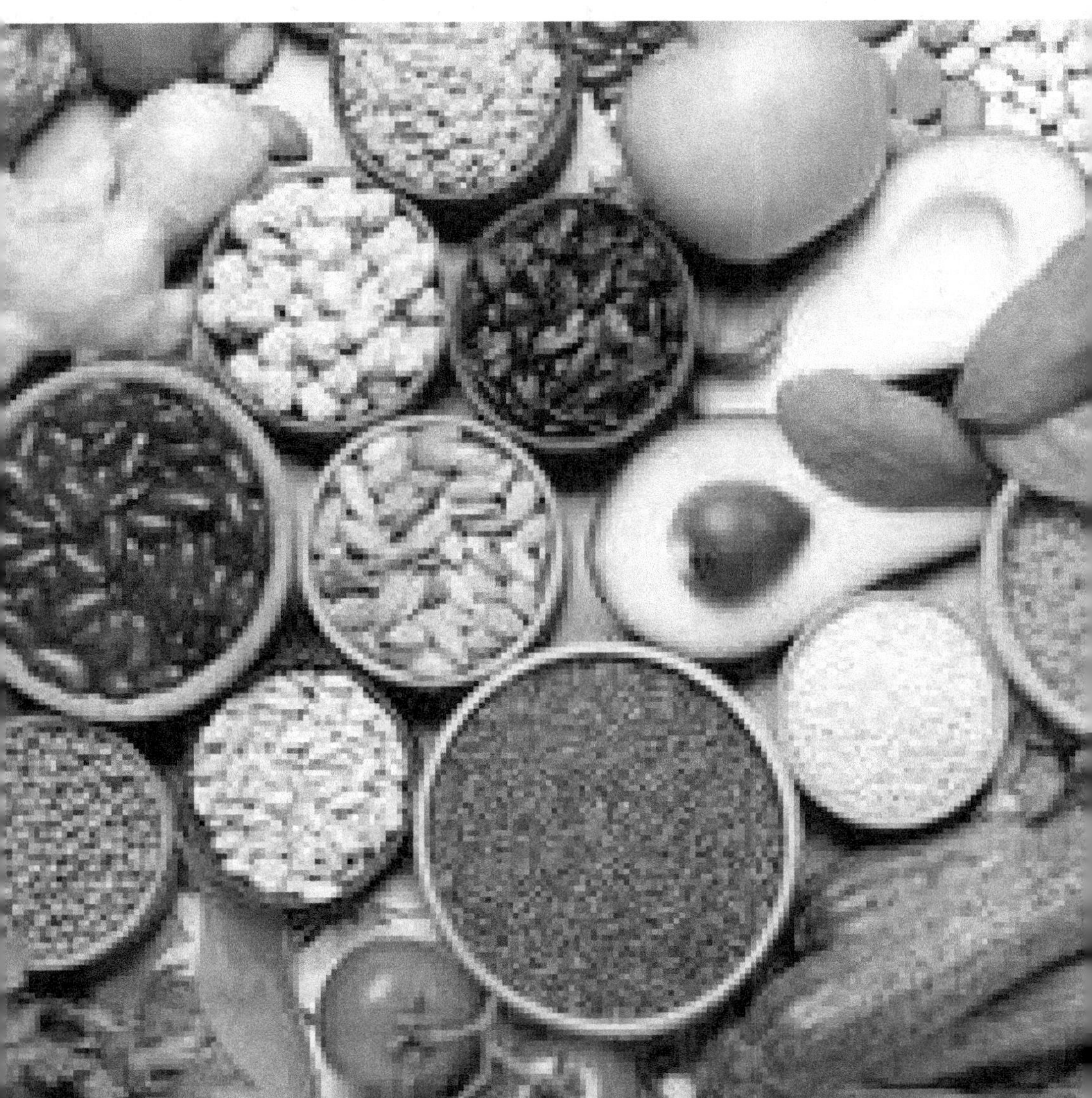

DISCLAIMER:

The information in this book should not be used to diagnose or treat any medical condition. Not every diet and exercise regimen are suitable for everyone.

Before beginning any diet, taking any medication, or beginning any fitness or weight-training program, you should always consult with a competent medical expert.

The author and publisher expressly disclaim all liability that may arise directly or indirectly from the use of this book. When using kitchen tools, operating ovens and burners, and handling raw food, always use common sense and safety precautions.

Readers are encouraged to seek professional assistance when necessary. This guide is provided for informational purposes only, and the author accepts no liability for any liabilities coming from the use of this information.

Printed in the United States of America.

First Edition: January 2024

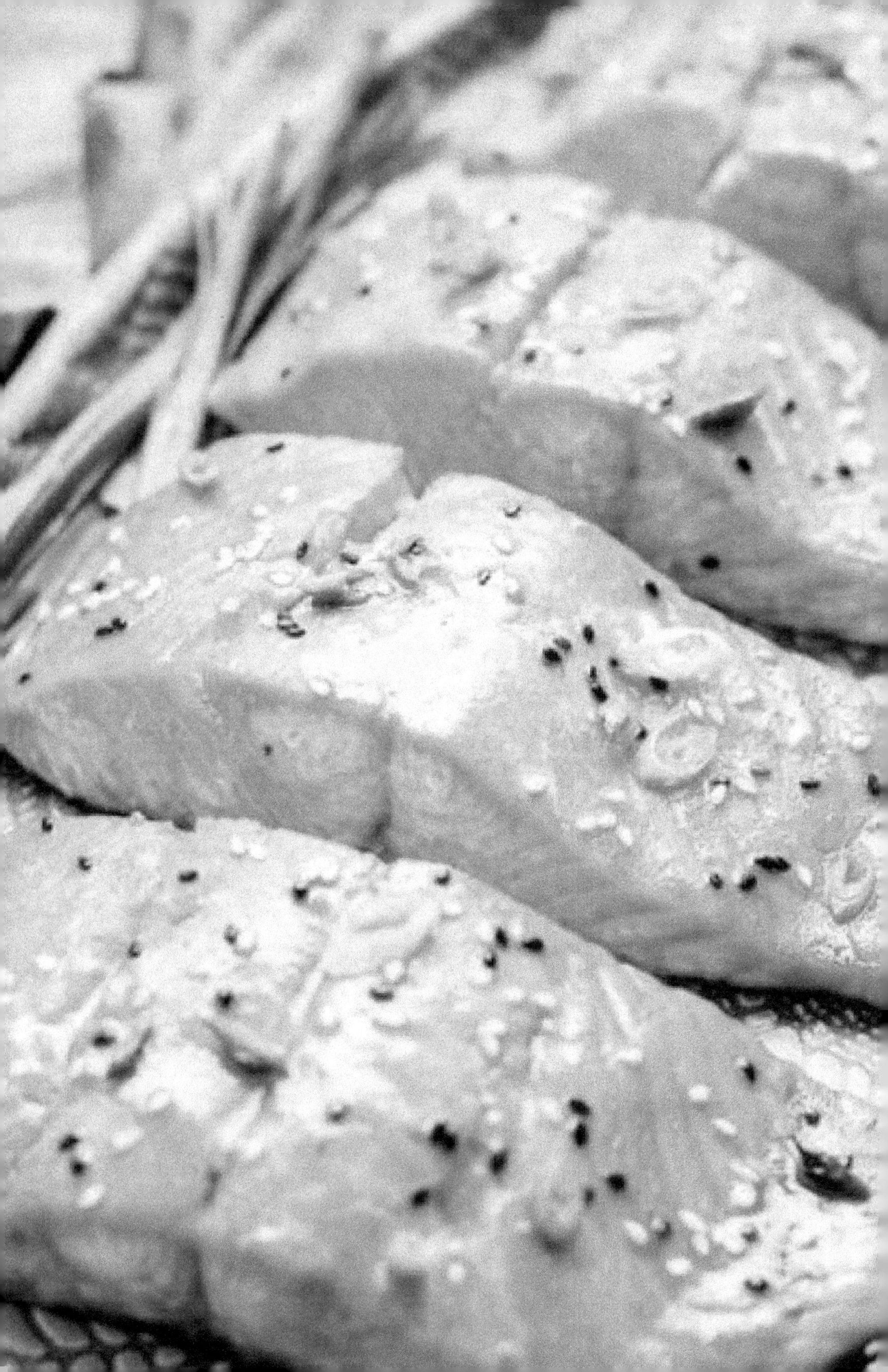

INTRODUCTION

In the pursuit of optimal health and wellness, the journey can be both challenging and rewarding. For individuals with an endomorphic body type, the struggle with a slow metabolism and the associated hurdles in losing weight can be particularly daunting. This comprehensive guide, "Metabolic Confusion Meal Plan for Endomorphs," is meticulously crafted to be your beacon of support, providing not just a roadmap but a transformative experience tailored specifically for individuals facing the unique challenges of slow metabolism.

1.1 Purpose of the Book

The purpose of this book is clear: to empower individuals with endomorphic body types with knowledge and strategies to harness the power of metabolic confusion for their benefit. We recognize the struggles faced by those dealing with a slow metabolism, and our aim is to offer not just information but a practical, actionable guide that facilitates a paradigm shift in how you approach nutrition, weight loss, and overall well-being.

As we delve into the intricacies of metabolic confusion, we'll navigate the science behind it, breaking down complex concepts into accessible and understandable information. This book is not merely a collection of theories; it's a practical resource, a companion on your journey to mastering your metabolism and achieving sustainable, long-term results.

1.2 Goals for the Reader

Embarking on this journey, it's crucial to establish tangible goals. These goals are not one-size-fits-all; they are crafted with your unique needs and aspirations in mind. Whether you're looking to shed excess weight, boost your metabolism, or simply adopt a healthier lifestyle, the goals set forth in this guide are designed to inspire and guide you towards success.

Through a holistic approach that combines nutritional guidance, strategic meal planning, and personalized strategies, our shared goal is to witness positive transformations in your body and overall well-being. The achievement of these goals is not just an endpoint but a continuous, evolving process that aligns with your individual journey toward a healthier, more vibrant you.

1.3 Brief Overview of Metabolic Confusion

At the heart of this guide lies the concept of metabolic confusion, a dynamic and effective approach to nutrition and weight management. The brief overview provided in this section serves as a foundational understanding of what metabolic confusion is, how it operates, and why it holds particular significance for individuals with endomorphic body types.

Metabolic confusion challenges traditional notions of dieting by introducing variety and adaptability. It involves strategically changing elements of your diet to keep the body guessing, preventing it from settling into a routine and thus optimizing metabolic processes. This section will unravel the complexities of metabolic confusion, bridging the gap between scientific principles and practical application.

As we proceed, we will delve deeper into the nuances of metabolic confusion, exploring its nuances and tailoring this approach to the specific needs of endomorphs. Through the exploration of strategic meal planning, personalized nutrition, and lifestyle adjustments, we aim to demystify metabolic confusion and make it a powerful tool in your journey toward improved health.

The pages that follow will be a comprehensive resource, offering not only knowledge but a step-by-step guide to implementing metabolic confusion for your benefit. Prepare to immerse yourself in a journey of discovery, empowerment, and transformation as we explore the world of "Metabolic Confusion Meal Plan for Endomorphs." Let the revolution in your health and well-being begin.

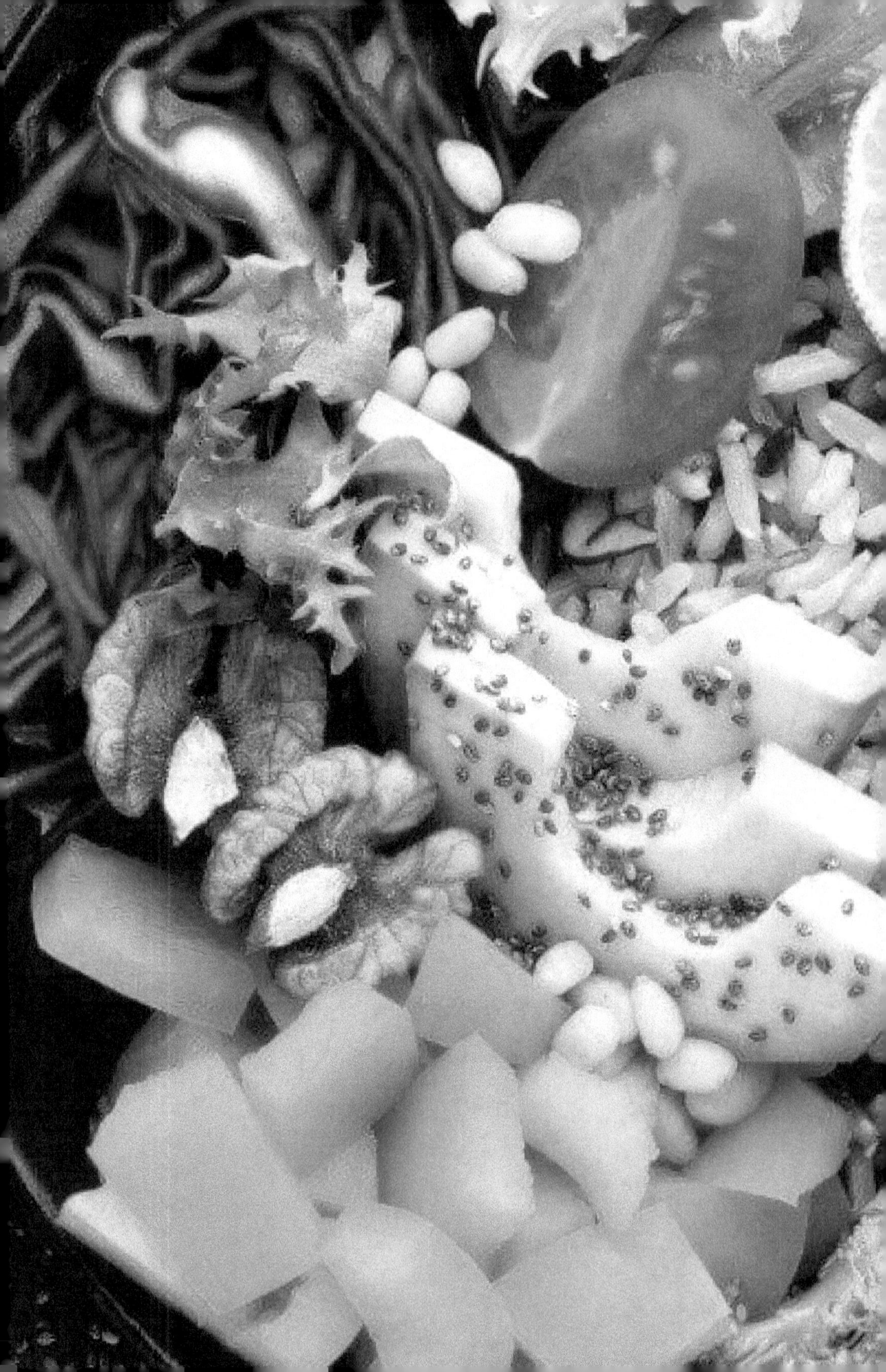

CHAPTER ONE
UNDERSTANDING YOUR BODY TYPE

1.1 Endomorph Characteristics

Endomorphs, as one of the three primary body types, exhibit distinctive physical and metabolic traits that set them apart on the spectrum of human anatomy. Characterized by a rounded physique with a higher proportion of body fat and a tendency to gain weight easily, endomorphs have a unique set of challenges and advantages in their journey toward health and fitness.

At the core of endomorph characteristics is a natural predisposition to store energy efficiently. This means that even with moderate calorie intake, endomorphs may find themselves grappling with weight management due to a slower metabolic rate. The body tends to preserve energy by storing excess calories as fat, particularly in areas like the abdomen and hips. Despite the challenges associated with this body type, endomorphs often possess a robust bone structure, which can contribute to a powerful and sturdy physique.

Understanding endomorph characteristics goes beyond superficial observations. It involves recognizing the body's inclination to develop a more extensive and curvier frame, often accompanied by a shorter stature. Endomorphs may also find themselves prone to a softer, rounder appearance compared to individuals with different body types.

Embracing your endomorphic characteristics requires a shift in mindset. Rather than viewing these traits as obstacles, consider them as unique features that contribute to your individuality. Your body type doesn't determine your destiny; it merely provides a starting point for a personalized approach to health and well-being.

1.2 Metabolism Challenges for Endomorphs

One of the primary challenges faced by endomorphs revolves around their metabolism, the intricate system responsible for converting food into energy. Endomorphs typically experience a slower metabolic rate, making it more challenging to burn calories efficiently. This predisposition toward a slower metabolism means that the body may hold onto calories rather than expending them, leading to weight gain and difficulty in shedding excess fat.

The metabolic challenges for endomorphs extend beyond the rate at which calories are burned; they also involve the body's response to different types of nutrients. Endomorphs may be more sensitive to carbohydrates, with a tendency to store them as fat rather than utilize them for energy. This unique metabolic response necessitates a thoughtful and individualized approach to nutrition.

Embracing the challenge of a slower metabolism involves adopting strategies that support metabolic health. This includes a focus on nutrient-dense foods, strategic meal timing, and incorporating physical activity that revs up the metabolism. Recognizing and addressing these challenges head-on is a crucial step in the journey toward optimal health for individuals with endomorphic body types.

1.3 Embracing Your Body Type

Embracing your endomorphic body type is not just an acceptance of your physical appearance; it's a commitment to understanding and working with your body's unique characteristics. It involves moving away from societal ideals and norms, recognizing that health and fitness are individual journeys shaped by personal factors, including genetics and body type.

The first step in embracing your body type is cultivating a positive self-image. Rather than fixating on perceived flaws, celebrate the strengths that come with being an endomorph. Focus on building a strong foundation that supports your overall well-being, including mental and emotional health.

Embracing your body type also involves adopting a tailored approach to nutrition and fitness. Recognize that your body may respond differently to certain foods and exercises compared to other body types. This understanding forms the basis for a personalized meal plan and workout routine that aligns with your goals and complements your unique physiology.

In the journey toward embracing your body type, surround yourself with positive influences. Seek support from communities that celebrate diversity in body shapes and sizes. Remember that health is a holistic concept that goes beyond external appearances, and by embracing your endomorphic body type, you embark on a path toward self-love, self-acceptance, and a fulfilling, sustainable approach to well-being.

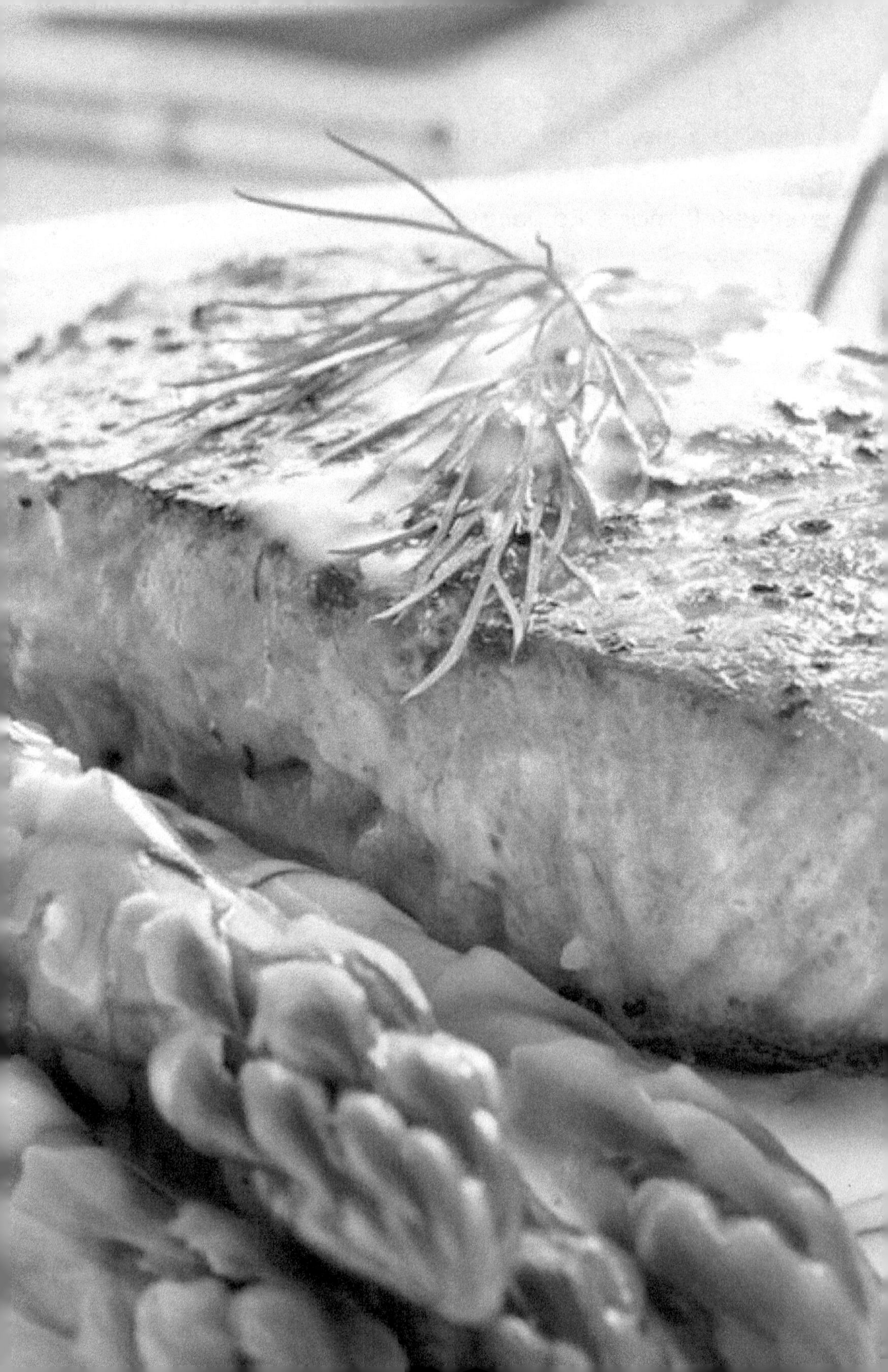

CHAPTER TWO
DEMYSTIFYING METABOLIC CONFUSION

2.1 What is Metabolic Confusion?

Metabolic confusion, a dynamic and innovative concept in the realm of nutrition and fitness, is a strategic approach aimed at keeping the body adaptable and responsive to dietary changes. At its core, metabolic confusion challenges the traditional idea of a static diet plan, advocating for variety and fluctuations in nutritional intake to prevent the body from settling into a routine. This approach recognizes the body's remarkable ability to adapt to consistent patterns, which can hinder progress in weight loss and overall metabolic health.

The essence of metabolic confusion lies in introducing controlled chaos into your dietary routine. Rather than adhering to a rigid and unchanging meal plan, individuals practicing metabolic confusion intentionally vary their calorie intake, macronutrient ratios, and meal timing. This variance prevents the body from adapting to a specific set of conditions, keeping it engaged and responsive to the nutritional stimuli it receives.

Implementing metabolic confusion doesn't imply randomness; it involves a structured and thoughtful approach to dietary changes. This may include cycling between high and low-calorie days, altering macronutrient distributions, and adjusting meal timings. The goal is to create an environment where the body is consistently challenged, leading to improved metabolic efficiency and enhanced fat-burning capabilities.

Understanding what metabolic confusion is also involves acknowledging its flexibility. This approach can be adapted to suit different dietary preferences, lifestyles, and body types. For endomorphs, the strategic application of metabolic confusion becomes particularly relevant, considering their unique metabolic challenges. By incorporating variety into their meal plans, endomorphs can disrupt stagnant metabolic patterns, potentially leading to more effective weight management.

2.2 How Metabolic Confusion Works

The mechanism behind metabolic confusion lies in its ability to prevent the body from settling into a metabolic plateau. When the body becomes accustomed to a consistent caloric intake and nutritional pattern, it adjusts its metabolic processes to become more efficient at handling those specific conditions. This adaptation can lead to a slowdown in metabolism, making it harder to burn calories and lose weight.

Metabolic confusion disrupts this adaptation process by introducing regular changes to the diet. This can involve altering the total caloric intake, adjusting the ratio of macronutrients (proteins, fats, and carbohydrates), and varying the timing of meals. By keeping the body guessing, metabolic confusion ensures that it doesn't optimize its processes for a specific set of conditions, thus promoting a more dynamic and responsive metabolism.

For endomorphs, whose bodies have a natural tendency to store excess calories as fat, the benefits of metabolic confusion are particularly significant. The strategic variations in dietary patterns prevent the body from clinging to calories, encouraging it to burn stored fat for energy. This not only aids in weight loss but also helps in overcoming the metabolic challenges associated with the endomorphic body type.

The cyclical nature of metabolic confusion aligns with the body's inherent adaptability. Just as muscles respond positively to varied workout routines, the metabolism benefits from a diverse range of nutritional stimuli. This variability not only prevents boredom in your diet but also promotes long-term adherence to healthy eating habits.

2.3 Benefits for Endomorphs

Endomorphs, with their predisposition to store energy efficiently and face challenges in weight management, can particularly benefit from the principles of metabolic confusion. The benefits extend beyond merely breaking weight loss plateaus; they encompass a holistic improvement in metabolic health and overall well-being.

Weight Management: One of the primary benefits for endomorphs is effective weight management. Metabolic confusion keeps the body from adapting to a specific caloric intake or nutritional pattern, preventing it from plateauing and promoting continuous fat burning. This can be especially advantageous for endomorphs looking to shed excess weight.

Optimized Fat Utilization: Metabolic confusion encourages the body to tap into its fat stores for energy. For endomorphs, whose bodies tend to store calories as fat, this can be a game-changer. By promoting the utilization of stored fat, metabolic confusion helps address the specific metabolic challenges faced by individuals with endomorphic body types.

Improved Metabolic Efficiency: The intentional variations in calorie intake and macronutrient distribution stimulate the metabolism, promoting adaptability and efficiency. This heightened metabolic activity can contribute to better overall energy expenditure, making it easier for endomorphs to achieve and maintain a healthy weight.

Sustained Motivation: The cyclical and dynamic nature of metabolic confusion adds an element of excitement and variety to the dietary routine. This can contribute to sustained motivation, making it more likely for individuals to adhere to their meal plans over the long term. Consistency is key in any wellness journey, and metabolic confusion offers a sustainable approach.

Balanced Hormones: Metabolic confusion can positively impact hormonal balance, a crucial factor in weight management. By avoiding prolonged periods of caloric restriction or excess, endomorphs can help regulate hormones responsible for hunger, satiety, and fat storage.

Embracing the benefits of metabolic confusion for endomorphs involves tailoring this approach to individual preferences, dietary requirements, and lifestyle factors. By incorporating strategic variations in their meal plans, endomorphs can unlock the full potential of their metabolism, leading to sustainable weight management and improved overall health.

CHAPTER THREE
TAILORING NUTRITION FOR ENDOMORPHS

3.1 Nutritional Needs of Endomorphs

Understanding the nutritional needs of endomorphs is a pivotal step in crafting an effective and sustainable meal plan. Endomorphs, with their propensity to store energy efficiently, have unique requirements that should be addressed to support their overall well-being and weight management goals.

One crucial aspect of the nutritional needs for endomorphs is a focus on nutrient-dense foods. These foods provide essential vitamins, minerals, and other beneficial compounds without excess calories. Whole grains, lean proteins, fruits, vegetables, and healthy fats form the foundation of a nutrient-dense diet for endomorphs. By prioritizing these foods, individuals can ensure they are meeting their nutritional requirements while managing their calorie intake.

Considering the potential sensitivity of endomorphs to carbohydrates, it becomes important to choose complex carbohydrates that offer sustained energy without causing drastic spikes in blood sugar levels. Opting for whole grains, legumes, and vegetables over refined carbohydrates can contribute to better blood sugar control and assist in weight management.

Another aspect of the nutritional needs for endomorphs is the importance of adequate protein intake. Protein plays a crucial role in muscle maintenance and repair, and it also contributes to a feeling of fullness, which can be beneficial for those aiming to manage their weight. Including lean protein sources such as poultry, fish, tofu, and legumes in each meal can support the unique needs of endomorphic bodies.

Balancing the nutritional needs of endomorphs also involves mindful portion control. While nutrient-dense foods are essential, it's crucial not to overconsume, as excess calories can contribute to weight gain. Learning to recognize hunger and fullness cues, practicing mindful eating, and avoiding emotional eating can all contribute to maintaining a healthy balance in caloric intake.

In summary, the nutritional needs of endomorphs revolve around choosing nutrient-dense foods, emphasizing complex carbohydrates, prioritizing lean protein sources, and practicing mindful portion control. Tailoring nutrition to suit the unique characteristics of endomorphic bodies sets the foundation for an effective meal plan that supports overall health and well-being.

3.2 Macronutrient Ratios

Macronutrient ratios play a pivotal role in tailoring nutrition for endomorphs. The distribution of macronutrients—carbohydrates, proteins, and fats—in the diet can have a significant impact on metabolism, energy levels, and weight management for individuals with endomorphic body types.

Carbohydrates:

Given the potential sensitivity of endomorphs to carbohydrates, it's essential to adopt a balanced and strategic approach. While carbohydrates are a primary energy source, focusing on complex carbohydrates with a lower glycemic index can help stabilize blood sugar levels and prevent energy crashes. Whole grains, legumes, and vegetables should be prioritized over refined carbohydrates. Additionally, incorporating carbohydrates earlier in the day when the body's metabolic rate tends to be higher can support energy needs.

Proteins:

Protein plays a crucial role in supporting muscle health, promoting a feeling of fullness, and aiding in weight management. Endomorphs benefit from a slightly higher protein intake, as it can contribute to the preservation of lean muscle mass and the burning of stored fat for energy. Including lean protein sources such as poultry, fish, eggs, and plant-based proteins in each meal helps maintain an optimal macronutrient balance.

Fats:

Dietary fats are an essential component of a balanced diet for endomorphs. Healthy fats, such as those found in avocados, nuts, seeds, and olive oil, provide a source of long-lasting energy and support overall well-being. Including a moderate amount of healthy fats in the diet not only enhances satiety but also aids in nutrient absorption. However, it's crucial to practice moderation, as fats are calorie-dense.

The ideal macronutrient ratio for endomorphs may vary based on individual factors such as activity level, metabolism, and personal preferences. Experimenting with different ratios and paying attention to how the body responds can help individuals find the balance that works best for them. It's also important to note that flexibility in macronutrient ratios can be beneficial, allowing for adjustments based on specific goals or changing dietary needs.

3.3 Timing and Frequency of Meals

The timing and frequency of meals play a significant role in optimizing metabolism and supporting weight management for endomorphs. Adopting a strategic approach to when and how often meals are consumed can contribute to stabilizing blood sugar levels, maintaining energy levels, and preventing overeating.

Regular Meal Timing:

Establishing a consistent meal timing routine is beneficial for endomorphs. Consuming meals and snacks at regular intervals throughout the day helps regulate blood sugar levels and prevents extreme fluctuations, which can contribute to cravings and overeating. Aim for three balanced meals and 1-2 snacks each day, spacing them evenly to provide a steady source of energy.

Breakfast Emphasis:

Front-loading caloric intake earlier in the day aligns with the body's natural circadian rhythm and can support metabolic efficiency. Breakfast, in particular, plays a crucial role in jumpstarting the metabolism after an overnight fast. Including a balanced combination of carbohydrates, proteins, and fats in the morning can set a positive tone for the rest of the day.

Nutrient Timing:

Strategic nutrient timing involves matching nutrient intake with the body's energy needs during different times of the day. For example, consuming a higher proportion of carbohydrates around workouts can provide the energy necessary for physical activity. Additionally, having a balanced meal or snack that includes protein before bedtime can support muscle repair and prevent overnight hunger.

Listening to Hunger Cues:

In addition to structured meal timing, it's essential to listen to hunger and fullness cues. Eating mindfully and paying attention to the body's signals can prevent overeating and promote a healthier relationship with food. Mindful eating involves savoring each bite, recognizing when full, and avoiding distractions during meals.

The timing and frequency of meals for endomorphs should involve regular, balanced meals and snacks, with an emphasis on breakfast and strategic nutrient timing. This approach supports stable blood sugar levels, sustained energy throughout the day, and optimal metabolic function. As with any aspect of nutrition, individual preferences and responses should guide the implementation of meal timing strategies for a personalized and effective approach.

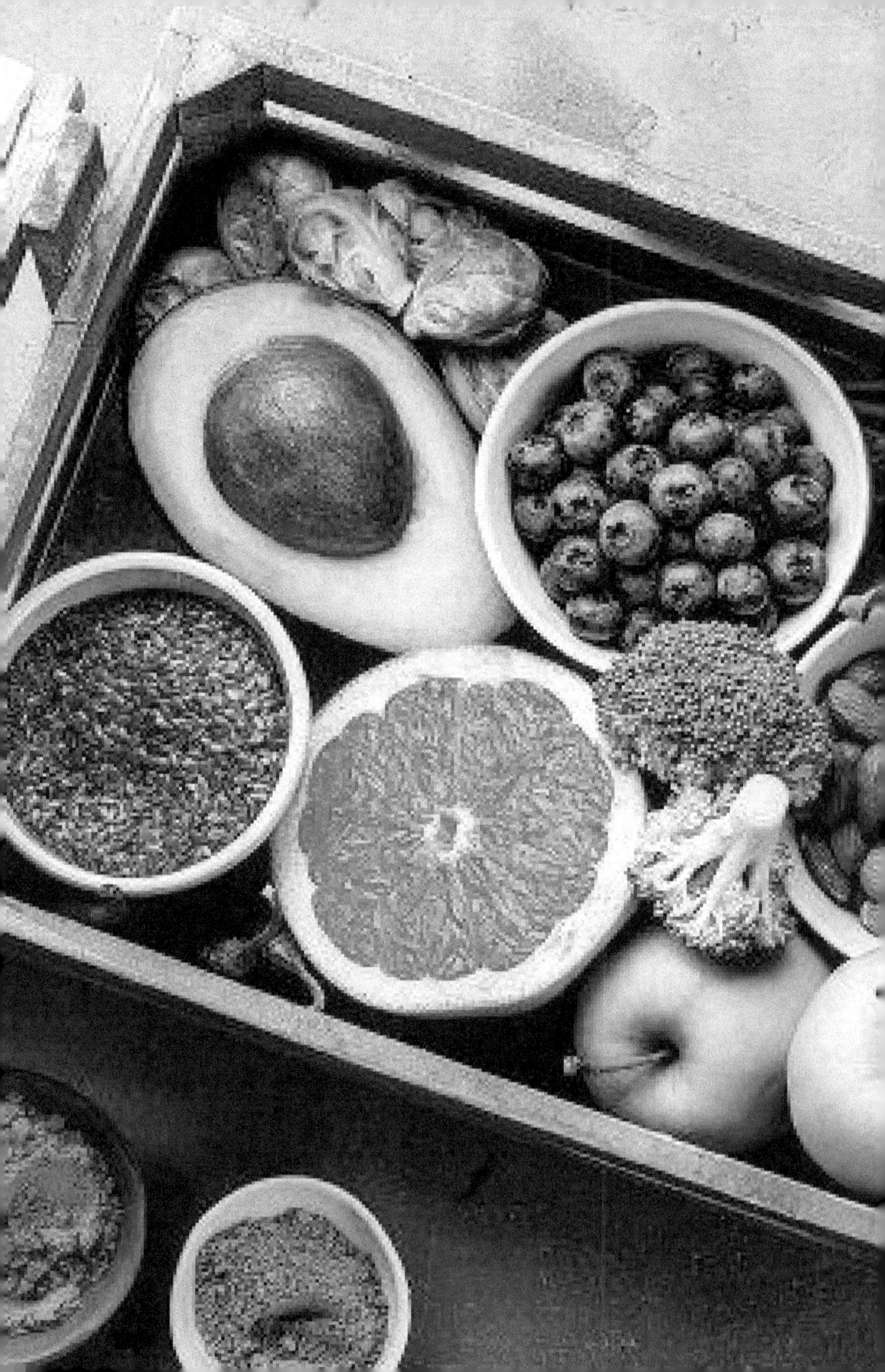

CHAPTER FOUR
CRAFTING YOUR METABOLIC CONFUSION MEAL PLAN

4.1 Building a Balanced Plate

Crafting a metabolic confusion meal plan starts with the foundation of a balanced plate. For endomorphs, the goal is to create meals that not only support nutritional needs but also strategically contribute to the principles of metabolic confusion. A balanced plate consists of a thoughtful combination of macronutrients and micronutrients, offering sustained energy and promoting optimal metabolic function.

Protein:

Begin by prioritizing a quality source of protein, a crucial component for endomorphs aiming for weight management. Protein not only supports muscle health but also contributes to a feeling of fullness. Opt for lean protein sources such as chicken, turkey, fish, tofu, legumes, and low-fat dairy products. Aim to include protein in each meal to provide a steady supply of amino acids and support metabolic processes.

Carbohydrates:

Incorporate complex carbohydrates to provide a steady release of energy and prevent blood sugar spikes. Whole grains like brown rice, quinoa, and oats, as well as starchy vegetables like sweet potatoes and legumes, are excellent choices. The fiber content in these carbohydrates supports digestive health and helps maintain a feeling of satiety, contributing to overall metabolic well-being.

Healthy Fats:

Include a moderate amount of healthy fats in your meal plan to support satiety and nutrient absorption. Avocados, nuts, seeds, olive oil, and fatty fish are rich sources of essential fatty acids. While fats are calorically dense, their inclusion in a balanced plate provides a sense of satisfaction and helps control appetite.

Vegetables and Fruits:

Load your plate with a variety of colorful vegetables and fruits to ensure a diverse range of essential vitamins and minerals. Vegetables are low in calories and high in fiber, contributing to the overall volume of your meal without significantly increasing caloric intake. This not only supports weight management but also enhances the nutritional value of your plate.

Hydration:

Don't forget the importance of hydration in building a balanced plate. Water is essential for metabolic processes, digestion, and overall well-being. Aim to include water-rich foods like fruits and vegetables in your meals and stay adequately hydrated throughout the day.

Building a balanced plate is about creating meals that are not only nutritionally rich but also aligned with the principles of metabolic confusion. By incorporating a variety of nutrients in each meal, endomorphs can foster an environment that keeps the body adaptable and responsive to dietary changes, promoting effective weight management.

4.2 Food Choices for Optimal Results

Choosing the right foods is pivotal when crafting a metabolic confusion meal plan for endomorphs. Optimal results come from selecting nutrient-dense, whole foods that align with the principles of metabolic confusion and address the specific needs of individuals with endomorphic body types.

Lean Proteins:

Lean protein sources should be a cornerstone of food choices for endomorphs. These proteins not only support muscle health but also contribute to metabolic efficiency. Opt for options such as poultry, fish, lean cuts of meat, tofu, and legumes. Including a variety of protein sources ensures a diverse amino acid profile, supporting overall metabolic function.

Complex Carbohydrates:

Prioritize complex carbohydrates to provide sustained energy and avoid rapid blood sugar fluctuations. Whole grains, including brown rice, quinoa, and whole wheat products, should feature prominently in the meal plan. Starchy vegetables like sweet potatoes and legumes are excellent choices, offering a mix of energy and essential nutrients.

Healthy Fats:

Incorporate healthy fats for satiety and overall well-being. Avocados, nuts, seeds, and olive oil are rich sources of monounsaturated and polyunsaturated fats. Including these fats in meals adds flavor, promotes satisfaction, and supports the absorption of fat-soluble vitamins.

Colorful Vegetables and Fruits:

Load up on a variety of colorful vegetables and fruits to maximize nutritional intake. These foods are rich in vitamins, minerals, and antioxidants, contributing to overall health. Incorporating a rainbow of produce ensures a diverse range of nutrients, supporting metabolic processes and promoting optimal well-being.

Water-Rich Foods:

Choose water-rich foods to enhance hydration. Vegetables and fruits with high water content, such as cucumbers, watermelon, and oranges, contribute to fluid intake and add volume to meals without significantly increasing caloric content. Hydration is essential for metabolic processes, and incorporating water-rich foods supports overall health.

Nutrient Timing:

Consider nutrient timing when making food choices. Strategically aligning nutrient intake with energy needs, such as consuming a balanced meal before workouts or prioritizing protein-rich foods after exercise, enhances the effectiveness of metabolic confusion. Tailoring food choices based on activity levels and timing can optimize results.

When selecting foods for optimal results in a metabolic confusion meal plan, variety is key. Diverse nutrient profiles not only contribute to overall health but also keep the body responsive to dietary changes, a fundamental aspect of metabolic confusion for endomorphs.

4.3 Meal Timing Strategies

Effective meal timing is a crucial component of a metabolic confusion meal plan for endomorphs. Strategic timing ensures that the body receives nutrients when it needs them most, supporting metabolic efficiency, energy levels, and weight management.

Breakfast Emphasis:

Front-load your caloric intake by emphasizing a nutritious breakfast. Breakfast plays a pivotal role in kickstarting the metabolism after an overnight fast. Including a mix of carbohydrates, proteins, and healthy fats provides a steady source of energy and sets a positive tone for the rest of the day.

Pre-Workout Nutrition:

Consider incorporating a balanced meal or snack before workouts to provide the energy necessary for physical activity. Including carbohydrates and a moderate amount of protein about 1-2 hours before exercise supports performance and contributes to the metabolic confusion principle.

Post-Workout Recovery:

Optimize post-workout recovery by consuming a meal or snack that includes protein and carbohydrates. This combination supports muscle repair, replenishes glycogen stores, and contributes to overall metabolic efficiency. Timing this meal within the post-exercise window enhances its effectiveness.

Balanced Meals and Snacks:

Space out meals and snacks evenly throughout the day to maintain steady blood sugar levels. Regular, balanced meals and snacks support metabolic function and prevent extreme fluctuations, reducing the likelihood of overeating during later meals.

Evening Nutrition:

Include a balanced meal or snack in the evening to support overnight recovery and prevent excessive hunger in the morning. Contrary to popular belief, eating in the evening does not inherently lead to weight gain. Instead, it can contribute to better overall nutrient distribution and support metabolic processes during rest.

Listen to Hunger Cues:

While strategic timing is important, it's equally crucial to listen to hunger and fullness cues. Pay attention to your body's signals, eat when hungry, and avoid restrictive practices. A mindful approach to meal timing promotes a healthy relationship with food and supports overall well-being.

Crafting a metabolic confusion meal plan involves not only selecting the right foods but also timing meals strategically. By aligning nutrient intake with the body's energy needs and incorporating balanced meals throughout the day, endomorphs can optimize the effectiveness of metabolic confusion, supporting their unique metabolic challenges and goals.

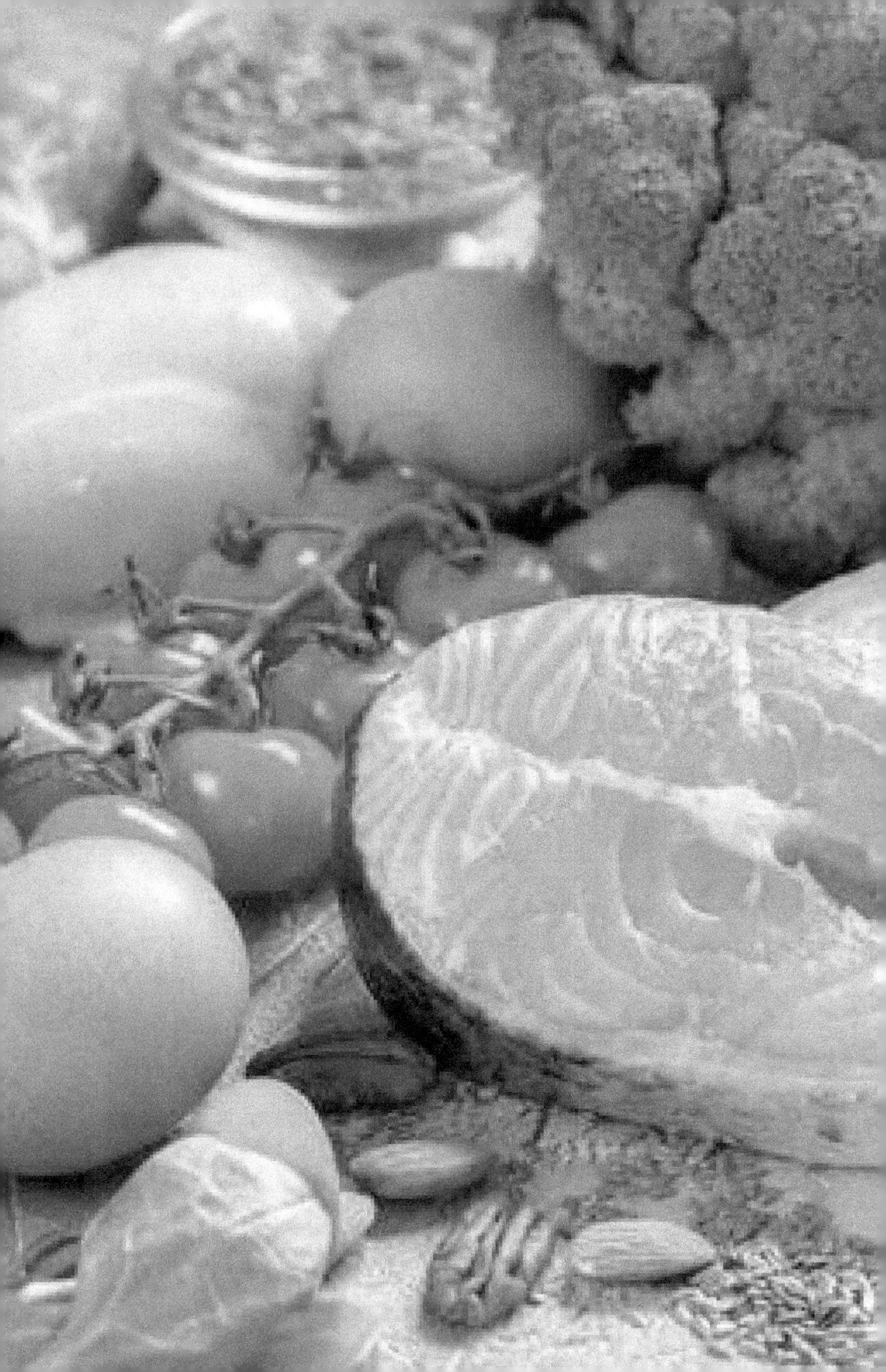

5.1 Weekday Meal Plans

Crafting a practical and effective metabolic confusion meal plan for weekdays requires a balance of variety, nutritional density, and simplicity. Weekdays often come with a busy schedule, making it crucial to have meal plans that are not only tailored to endomorphic needs but also convenient to prepare and consume.

Day 1:

- **Breakfast:** Scrambled eggs with spinach and whole-grain toast

- **Mid-Morning Snack:** Greek yogurt with berries

- **Lunch:** Grilled chicken salad with mixed vegetables and quinoa

- **Afternoon Snack:** Handful of almonds with an apple

- **Dinner:** Baked salmon with sweet potato and steamed broccoli

Day 2:

- **Breakfast:** Oatmeal with sliced banana and a sprinkle of chia seeds

- **Mid-Morning Snack:** Cottage cheese with pineapple chunks

- **Lunch:** Turkey and avocado wrap with whole-grain tortilla

- **Afternoon Snack:** Carrot sticks with hummus

- **Dinner:** Stir-fried tofu with brown rice and mixed vegetables

Day 3:

- **Breakfast:** Whole-grain pancakes with Greek yogurt and berries
- **Mid-Morning Snack:** Handful of walnuts with a pear
- **Lunch:** Quinoa bowl with black beans, corn, tomatoes, and avocado
- **Afternoon Snack:** Cottage cheese with sliced strawberries
- **Dinner:** Grilled shrimp with quinoa and roasted Brussels sprouts

Day 4:

- **Breakfast:**
    - Scrambled eggs with spinach and whole-grain toast
- **Mid-Morning Snack:**
    - Greek yogurt with mixed berries
- **Lunch:**
    - Grilled chicken salad with mixed greens, cherry tomatoes, cucumber, and quinoa
- **Afternoon Snack:**
    - Handful of almonds with an apple
- **Dinner:**
    - Baked salmon with sweet potato and steamed broccoli

Day 5:

- **Breakfast:**
    - Overnight oats with sliced banana and a sprinkle of chia seeds
- **Mid-Morning Snack:**
    - Cottage cheese with pineapple chunks
- **Lunch:**
    - Turkey and avocado wrap with whole-grain tortilla
- **Afternoon Snack:**
    - Carrot sticks with hummus
- **Dinner:**
    - Stir-fried tofu with brown rice and mixed vegetables

Day 6:

- **Breakfast:**
    - Whole-grain pancakes with Greek yogurt and mixed berries
- **Mid-Morning Snack:**
    - Handful of walnuts with a pear
- **Lunch:**
    - Quinoa bowl with black beans, corn, tomatoes, and avocado
- **Afternoon Snack:**
    - Cottage cheese with sliced strawberries

- **Dinner:**
    - Grilled shrimp with quinoa and roasted Brussels sprouts

Day 7:

- **Breakfast:**
    - Green smoothie with spinach, banana, and protein powder
- **Mid-Morning Snack:**
    - Whole-grain crackers with cheese
- **Lunch:**
    - Chicken and vegetable stir-fry with brown rice
- **Afternoon Snack:**
    - Greek yogurt with a drizzle of honey
- **Dinner:**
    - Baked cod with sweet potato wedges and steamed asparagus

Day 8:

- **Breakfast:**
    - Avocado toast with poached eggs on whole-grain bread
- **Mid-Morning Snack:**
    - Mixed nuts with dried fruits
- **Lunch:**
    - Lentil soup with a side of whole-grain bread

- **Afternoon Snack:**
    - Sliced cucumber with hummus
- **Dinner:**
    - Grilled chicken breast with quinoa and roasted vegetables

Day 9:

- **Breakfast:**
    - Chia seed pudding with almond milk and fresh berries
- **Mid-Morning Snack:**
    - Apple slices with peanut butter
- **Lunch:**
    - Spinach and feta-stuffed chicken breast with quinoa
- **Afternoon Snack:**
    - Cottage cheese with sliced peaches
- **Dinner:**
    - Baked turkey meatballs with whole-grain spaghetti and tomato sauce

Day 10:

- **Breakfast:**
    - Whole-grain waffles with Greek yogurt and sliced strawberries
- **Mid-Morning Snack:**
    - Trail mix with a mix of nuts and dried fruits

- **Lunch:**
    - Chickpea salad with mixed vegetables, feta cheese, and olive oil dressing
- **Afternoon Snack:**
    - Celery sticks with cream cheese
- **Dinner:**
    - Grilled salmon with quinoa and steamed broccoli

Day 11:

- **Breakfast:**
    - Spinach and feta omelette with whole-grain toast
- **Mid-Morning Snack:**
    - Greek yogurt parfait with granola and mixed berries
- **Lunch:**
    - Quinoa salad with grilled chicken, cherry tomatoes, cucumbers, and a lemon vinaigrette
- **Afternoon Snack:**
    - Sliced bell peppers with hummus
- **Dinner:**
    - Baked cod with sweet potato wedges and steamed broccoli

Day 12:

- **Breakfast:**
    - Overnight chia seed pudding with almond milk and sliced mango
- **Mid-Morning Snack:**
    - Apple slices with peanut butter
- **Lunch:**
    - Turkey and avocado wrap with whole-grain tortilla
- **Afternoon Snack:**
    - Mixed nuts with dried fruits
- **Dinner:**
    - Stir-fried tofu with quinoa and mixed vegetables

Day 13:

- **Breakfast:**
    - Whole-grain pancakes with Greek yogurt and blueberries
- **Mid-Morning Snack:**
    - Cottage cheese with pineapple chunks
- **Lunch:**
    - Lentil soup with a side of whole-grain bread
- **Afternoon Snack:**
    - Carrot sticks with hummus

- **Dinner:**

    - Grilled shrimp with brown rice and roasted Brussels sprouts

Day 14:

- **Breakfast:**

    - Avocado toast with poached eggs on whole-grain bread

- **Mid-Morning Snack:**

    - Trail mix with a mix of nuts and seeds

- **Lunch:**

    - Chickpea salad with mixed vegetables, feta cheese, and olive oil dressing

- **Afternoon Snack:**

    - Sliced cucumber with tzatziki

- **Dinner:**

    - Baked chicken breast with quinoa and steamed asparagus

Day 15:

- **Breakfast:**

    - Berry and banana smoothie with spinach and protein powder

- **Mid-Morning Snack:**

    - Handful of almonds with an orange

- **Lunch:**

    - Spinach and feta-stuffed chicken breast with quinoa

- **Afternoon Snack:**
    - Greek yogurt with a drizzle of honey
- **Dinner:**
    - Grilled salmon with sweet potato and steamed green beans

Day 16:

- **Breakfast:**
    - Whole-grain waffles with Greek yogurt and sliced strawberries
- **Mid-Morning Snack:**
    - Celery sticks with cream cheese
- **Lunch:**
    - Quinoa bowl with black beans, corn, tomatoes, and avocado
- **Afternoon Snack:**
    - Cottage cheese with sliced peaches
- **Dinner:**
    - Baked turkey meatballs with whole-grain spaghetti and tomato sauce

Day 17:

- **Breakfast:**
    - Scrambled eggs with sautéed spinach and whole-grain toast
- **Mid-Morning Snack:**
    - Banana slices with almond butter

- **Lunch:**
    - Grilled chicken salad with mixed greens, cherry tomatoes, cucumber, and quinoa
- **Afternoon Snack:**
    - Sliced bell peppers with hummus
- **Dinner:**
    - Stir-fried tofu with brown rice and mixed vegetables

Day 18:

- **Breakfast:**
    - Oatmeal with sliced banana, chia seeds, and a dollop of yogurt
- **Mid-Morning Snack:**
    - Mixed nuts with dried fruits
- **Lunch:**
    - Turkey and avocado wrap with whole-grain tortilla
- **Afternoon Snack:**
    - Apple slices with peanut butter
- **Dinner:**
    - Baked cod with quinoa and roasted Brussels sprouts

Day 19:

- **Breakfast:**

    - Whole-grain pancakes with Greek yogurt and mixed berries

- **Mid-Morning Snack:**

    - Cottage cheese with pineapple chunks

- **Lunch:**

    - Lentil soup with a side of whole-grain bread

- **Afternoon Snack:**

    - Carrot sticks with hummus

- **Dinner:**

    - Grilled shrimp with brown rice and steamed green beans

Day 20:

- **Breakfast:**

    - Avocado toast with poached eggs on whole-grain bread

- **Mid-Morning Snack:**

    - Trail mix with a mix of nuts and seeds

- **Lunch:**

    - Chickpea salad with mixed vegetables, feta cheese, and olive oil dressing

- **Afternoon Snack:**

    - Sliced cucumber with tzatziki

- **Dinner:**

    - Baked chicken breast with quinoa and steamed asparagus

Day 21:

- **Breakfast:**

    - Scrambled eggs with spinach and whole-grain toast

- **Mid-Morning Snack:**

    - Greek yogurt with mixed berries

- **Lunch:**

    - Grilled chicken salad with mixed greens, cherry tomatoes, cucumber, and quinoa

- **Afternoon Snack:**

    - Handful of almonds with an apple

- **Dinner:**

    - Baked cod with sweet potato wedges and steamed broccoli

Day 22:

- **Breakfast:**

    - Overnight chia seed pudding with almond milk and sliced mango

- **Mid-Morning Snack:**

    - Apple slices with peanut butter

- **Lunch:**

    - Turkey and avocado wrap with whole-grain tortilla

- **Afternoon Snack:**
    - Mixed nuts with dried fruits
- **Dinner:**
    - Stir-fried tofu with quinoa and mixed vegetables

Day 23:

- **Breakfast:**
    - Whole-grain pancakes with Greek yogurt and blueberries
- **Mid-Morning Snack:**
    - Cottage cheese with pineapple chunks
- **Lunch:**
    - Lentil soup with a side of whole-grain bread
- **Afternoon Snack:**
    - Carrot sticks with hummus
- **Dinner:**
    - Grilled shrimp with brown rice and roasted Brussels sprouts

Day 24:

- **Breakfast:**
    - Avocado toast with poached eggs on whole-grain bread
- **Mid-Morning Snack:**
    - Trail mix with a mix of nuts and seeds

- **Lunch:**
    - Chickpea salad with mixed vegetables, feta cheese, and olive oil dressing
- **Afternoon Snack:**
    - Sliced cucumber with tzatziki
- **Dinner:**
    - Baked chicken breast with quinoa and steamed asparagus

Day 25:

- **Breakfast:**
    - Berry and banana smoothie with spinach and protein powder
- **Mid-Morning Snack:**
    - Handful of almonds with an orange
- **Lunch:**
    - Spinach and feta-stuffed chicken breast with quinoa
- **Afternoon Snack:**
    - Greek yogurt with a drizzle of honey
- **Dinner:**
    - Grilled salmon with sweet potato and steamed green beans

Day 26:

- **Breakfast:**
    - Whole-grain waffles with Greek yogurt and sliced strawberries
- **Mid-Morning Snack:**
    - Celery sticks with cream cheese
- **Lunch:**
    - Quinoa bowl with black beans, corn, tomatoes, and avocado
- **Afternoon Snack:**
    - Cottage cheese with sliced peaches
- **Dinner:**
    - Baked turkey meatballs with whole-grain spaghetti and tomato sauce

Day 27:

- **Breakfast:**
    - Scrambled eggs with sautéed spinach and whole-grain toast
- **Mid-Morning Snack:**
    - Banana slices with almond butter
- **Lunch:**
    - Grilled chicken salad with mixed greens, cherry tomatoes, cucumber, and quinoa

- **Afternoon Snack:**

    - Sliced bell peppers with hummus

- **Dinner:**

    - Stir-fried tofu with brown rice and mixed vegetables

Day 28:

- **Breakfast:**

    - Oatmeal with sliced banana, chia seeds, and a dollop of yogurt

- **Mid-Morning Snack:**

    - Mixed nuts with dried fruits

- **Lunch:**

    - Turkey and avocado wrap with whole-grain tortilla

- **Afternoon Snack:**

    - Apple slices with peanut butter

- **Dinner:**

    - Baked cod with quinoa and roasted Brussels sprouts

These weekday meal plans are designed to be flexible, allowing for easy adaptation based on individual preferences and dietary requirements. The key is to ensure a balance of macronutrients, incorporate a variety of nutrient-dense foods, and maintain portion control for effective metabolic confusion throughout the week.

5.2 Weekend Specials

Weekends present an opportunity to indulge in slightly more elaborate and enjoyable meals while still adhering to the principles of metabolic confusion. These weekend specials can add excitement to the meal plan without compromising on health and nutrition.

Saturday Brunch:

- **Avocado Toast with Poached Eggs:** Whole-grain toast topped with mashed avocado and poached eggs, sprinkled with chili flakes.

- **Mixed Berry Smoothie:** A blend of assorted berries, Greek yogurt, and a splash of almond milk.

Sunday Dinner:

- **Grilled Steak with Chimichurri Sauce:** Lean beef steak marinated and grilled, served with a vibrant chimichurri sauce.

- **Quinoa and Roasted Vegetable Salad:** Quinoa mixed with roasted zucchini, bell peppers, cherry tomatoes, and feta cheese.

Weekend Dessert:

- **Dark Chocolate-Dipped Strawberries:** Fresh strawberries dipped in melted dark chocolate, chilled until the chocolate hardens.

Saturday Brunch:

- **1. Avocado and Smoked Salmon Bagel:**

  - Toasted whole-grain bagel topped with creamy avocado slices and smoked salmon. Garnish with fresh dill and a squeeze of lemon.

- **2. Greek Yogurt Parfait:**
  - Layer Greek yogurt with granola, mixed berries, and a drizzle of honey for a delightful and indulgent parfait.

Saturday Dinner:

- **3. Grilled Steak with Mushroom Sauce:**
  - Juicy grilled steak served with a rich mushroom sauce. Pair it with roasted sweet potatoes and sautéed green beans.

- **4. Shrimp and Asparagus Risotto:**
  - Creamy risotto made with Arborio rice, succulent shrimp, and crisp asparagus. Finish with a sprinkle of Parmesan cheese.

Sunday Brunch:

- **5. Blueberry Ricotta Pancakes:**
  - Fluffy pancakes made with ricotta cheese and studded with fresh blueberries. Serve with a dollop of Greek yogurt and a drizzle of maple syrup.

- **6. Smashed Avocado and Poached Egg Toast:**
  - Rustic whole-grain toast topped with smashed avocado, a perfectly poached egg, and a sprinkle of red pepper flakes.

Sunday Dinner:

- **7. Lemon Garlic Herb Roast Chicken:**
  - Whole roast chicken seasoned with lemon, garlic, and fresh herbs. Accompany with roasted Brussels sprouts and quinoa.

- **8. Baked Cod with Mango Salsa:**

    - Light and flavorful baked cod topped with a refreshing mango salsa. Serve with cilantro-lime rice for a tropical twist.

Weekend Desserts:

- **9. Dark Chocolate Avocado Mousse:**

    - Decadent chocolate mousse made with ripe avocados, dark chocolate, and a touch of maple syrup. Chill for a velvety dessert.

- **10. Mixed Berry Crumble:**

    - Baked mixed berries topped with a wholesome crumble made from oats, almond flour, and a hint of cinnamon. Serve warm with a scoop of vanilla Greek yogurt.

Including weekend specials adds a touch of variety and culinary enjoyment to the metabolic confusion meal plan. While these meals may be slightly more indulgent, they still adhere to the principles of balanced nutrition and portion control.

5.3 Quick and Easy Recipes For Busy Days

On busy days, having quick and easy recipes that align with the principles of metabolic confusion is essential. These recipes prioritize simplicity without compromising on taste or nutritional value.

Here are 50 quick and easy recipes that align with the principles of metabolic confusion, focusing on simplicity, taste, and nutritional value. Please note that the nutritional information provided is approximate and may vary based on specific ingredients and portion sizes.

1. Quick Stir-Fry:

Ingredients:

- Lean protein (chicken, tofu, or shrimp)
- Mixed vegetables (broccoli, bell peppers, snap peas)
- Soy sauce, garlic, ginger for seasoning
- Brown rice or quinoa for serving

Instructions:

1. Stir-fry the chosen protein and vegetables in a pan with soy sauce, garlic, and ginger.
2. Serve over a bed of brown rice or quinoa.

Nutritional Information:

- Calories: 350-450 per serving
- Protein: 25-30g
- Carbohydrates: 40-50g
- Fat: 10-15g

2. Mediterranean Chickpea Salad:

Ingredients:

- Canned chickpeas, rinsed and drained
- Cherry tomatoes, cucumber, red onion, chopped
- Feta cheese, crumbled
- Olive oil, lemon juice, oregano for dressing

Instructions:

1. Combine chickpeas, vegetables, and feta in a bowl.
2. Whisk together olive oil, lemon juice, and oregano for the dressing.
3. Toss the salad with the dressing and enjoy.

Nutritional Information:

- Calories: 300-400 per serving
- Protein: 10-15g
- Carbohydrates: 30-40g
- Fat: 15-20g

3. 10-Minute Breakfast Smoothie:

Ingredients:

- Spinach, banana, and frozen berries
- Greek yogurt or almond milk
- Chia seeds or flaxseeds

Instructions:

1. Blend spinach, banana, berries, and yogurt or almond milk.
2. Add chia seeds or flaxseeds for an extra nutritional boost.

Nutritional Information:

- Calories: 250-350 per serving
- Protein: 15-20g
- Carbohydrates: 30-40g
- Fat: 10-15g

4. Quick Quinoa Bowl:

Ingredients:

- Cooked quinoa
- Black beans, corn, cherry tomatoes, avocado
- Lime juice, cilantro for flavor

Instructions:

1. Mix quinoa with black beans, corn, tomatoes, and avocado.
2. Drizzle with lime juice and garnish with cilantro.

Nutritional Information:

- Calories: 300-400 per serving
- Protein: 10-15g
- Carbohydrates: 40-50g
- Fat: 10-15g

5. Caprese Chicken Skillet:

Ingredients:

- Chicken breast
- Cherry tomatoes, mozzarella, basil
- Balsamic glaze for drizzling

Instructions:

1. Cook chicken in a skillet, top with cherry tomatoes, mozzarella, and basil.
2. Drizzle with balsamic glaze before serving.

Nutritional Information:

- Calories: 350-450 per serving
- Protein: 30-35g
- Carbohydrates: 5-10g
- Fat: 15-20g

6. Sweet Potato and Chickpea Curry:

Ingredients:

- Sweet potatoes, chickpeas, spinach
- Coconut milk, curry paste, turmeric
- Brown rice for serving

Instructions:

1. Cook sweet potatoes, chickpeas, and spinach in a curry sauce.
2. Serve over brown rice.

Nutritional Information:

- Calories: 400-500 per serving
- Protein: 15-20g
- Carbohydrates: 50-60g
- Fat: 15-20g

7. Turkey and Quinoa Stuffed Peppers:

Ingredients:

- Ground turkey, quinoa, bell peppers
- Tomato sauce, black beans, corn
- Mexican seasoning for flavor

Instructions:

1. Cook turkey and quinoa, mix with black beans, corn, and seasoning.
2. Stuff into halved bell peppers and bake.

Nutritional Information:

- Calories: 350-450 per serving
- Protein: 25-30g

- Carbohydrates: 30-40g

- Fat: 10-15g

8. Veggie-Packed Omelette:

Ingredients:

- Eggs, spinach, tomatoes, mushrooms

- Feta cheese, herbs for flavor

Instructions:

1. Whisk eggs and pour into a pan with spinach, tomatoes, and mushrooms.

2. Add feta and herbs before folding.

Nutritional Information:

- Calories: 250-350 per serving

- Protein: 15-20g

- Carbohydrates: 5-10g

- Fat: 15-20g

9. Grilled Salmon with Quinoa Salad:

Ingredients:

- Salmon fillet

- Quinoa, cucumber, cherry tomatoes

- Lemon, dill for dressing

Instructions:

1. Grill salmon and serve over a quinoa salad.

2. Dress with lemon and dill.

Nutritional Information:

- Calories: 400-500 per serving
- Protein: 30-35g
- Carbohydrates: 30-40g
- Fat: 15-20g

10. Zucchini Noodles with Pesto and Shrimp:

Ingredients:

- Zucchini noodles
- Shrimp, cherry tomatoes, pine nuts
- Pesto sauce for flavor

Instructions:

1. Saute shrimp, cherry tomatoes, and pine nuts.
2. Toss with zucchini noodles and pesto sauce.

Nutritional Information:

- Calories: 300-400 per serving
- Protein: 20-25g
- Carbohydrates: 15-20g
- Fat: 15-20g

11. Shrimp and Quinoa Stir-Fry:

Ingredients:

- Shrimp, cooked quinoa, mixed vegetables
- Soy sauce, garlic, ginger for seasoning

Instructions:

1. Stir-fry shrimp and mixed vegetables in a pan with soy sauce, garlic, and ginger.

2. Mix in cooked quinoa.

Nutritional Information:

- Calories: 300-400 per serving
- Protein: 20-25g
- Carbohydrates: 30-40g
- Fat: 10-15g

12. Mediterranean Stuffed Bell Peppers:

Ingredients:

- Ground turkey, cooked quinoa, cherry tomatoes, feta
- Kalamata olives, oregano for flavor

Instructions:

1. Brown ground turkey and mix with cooked quinoa, cherry tomatoes, feta, olives, and oregano.
2. Stuff the mixture into halved bell peppers and bake.

Nutritional Information:

- Calories: 350-450 per serving
- Protein: 25-30g
- Carbohydrates: 30-40g
- Fat: 15-20g

13. Caprese Quinoa Salad:

Ingredients:

- Cooked quinoa, cherry tomatoes, mozzarella, basil
- Balsamic glaze for drizzling

Instructions:

1. Combine quinoa, cherry tomatoes, mozzarella, and basil.
2. Drizzle with balsamic glaze before serving.

Nutritional Information:

- Calories: 300-400 per serving
- Protein: 10-15g
- Carbohydrates: 30-40g
- Fat: 15-20g

14. Teriyaki Chicken Lettuce Wraps:

Ingredients:

- Grilled chicken, water chestnuts, bell peppers
- Teriyaki sauce, lettuce leaves

Instructions:

1. Mix grilled chicken, water chestnuts, and bell peppers with teriyaki sauce.
2. Spoon the mixture into lettuce leaves for wraps.

Nutritional Information:

- Calories: 250-350 per serving
- Protein: 20-25g
- Carbohydrates: 15-20g
- Fat: 10-15g

15. Cauliflower Fried Rice:

Ingredients:

- Cauliflower rice, mixed vegetables, egg
- Soy sauce, sesame oil, green onions for seasoning

Instructions:

1. Saute cauliflower rice, mixed vegetables, and scrambled egg with soy sauce, sesame oil, and green onions.

Nutritional Information:

- Calories: 200-300 per serving
- Protein: 10-15g
- Carbohydrates: 20-30g
- Fat: 10-15g

16. Lemon Garlic Shrimp Pasta:

Ingredients:

- Shrimp, whole-grain spaghetti, cherry tomatoes
- Garlic, lemon, parsley for flavor

Instructions:

1. Cook shrimp and whole-grain spaghetti. Toss with cherry tomatoes, garlic, lemon, and parsley.

Nutritional Information:

- Calories: 350-450 per serving
- Protein: 25-30g
- Carbohydrates: 40-50g
- Fat: 10-15g

17. Turkey and Vegetable Skewers:

Ingredients:

- Turkey cubes, bell peppers, red onion
- Olive oil, rosemary, lemon for marinating

Instructions:

1. Marinate turkey cubes, bell peppers, and red onion in olive oil, rosemary, and lemon.

2. Skewer and grill until cooked.

Nutritional Information:

- Calories: 300-400 per serving
- Protein: 25-30g
- Carbohydrates: 10-15g
- Fat: 15-20g

18. Black Bean and Corn Salad:

Ingredients:

- Black beans, corn, cherry tomatoes, red onion
- Lime juice, cilantro for dressing

Instructions:

1. Mix black beans, corn, cherry tomatoes, and red onion.

2. Dress with lime juice and cilantro.

Nutritional Information:

- Calories: 250-350 per serving
- Protein: 10-15g
- Carbohydrates: 40-50g
- Fat: 5-10g

19. Eggplant and Chickpea Curry:

Ingredients:

- Eggplant, chickpeas, spinach
- Coconut milk, curry paste, turmeric

Instructions:

1. Cook eggplant, chickpeas, and spinach in a curry sauce with coconut milk, curry paste, and turmeric.

2. Serve over brown rice.

Nutritional Information:

- Calories: 350-450 per serving
- Protein: 15-20g
- Carbohydrates: 40-50g / Fat: 15-20g

20. Spinach and Feta Stuffed Chicken Breast:

Ingredients:

- Chicken breast, spinach, feta cheese
- Garlic, lemon, herbs for seasoning

Instructions:

1. Season chicken breast and stuff with a mixture of spinach and feta.

2. Bake until chicken is cooked through.

Nutritional Information:

- Calories: 300-400 per serving
- Protein: 30-35g
- Carbohydrates: 5-10g
- Fat: 15-20g

Ingredients:

- Cooked quinoa, black beans, corn, diced tomatoes
- Avocado, lime, cilantro for garnish

Instructions:

1. Mix quinoa, black beans, corn, and diced tomatoes in a bowl.
2. Top with sliced avocado, a squeeze of lime, and fresh cilantro.

Nutritional Information:

- Calories: 300-400 per serving
- Protein: 15-20g
- Carbohydrates: 40-50g
- Fat: 10-15g

Ingredients:

- Cod fillets, lemon, garlic, fresh herbs
- Olive oil, salt, and pepper

Instructions:

1. Marinate cod in olive oil, lemon, garlic, and fresh herbs.
2. Bake until the fish is cooked through and flakes easily.

Nutritional Information:

- Calories: 250-350 per serving
- Protein: 30-35g
- Carbohydrates: 5-10g

- Fat: 15-20g

23. Chickpea and Vegetable Stir-Fry:

Ingredients:

- Chickpeas, broccoli, bell peppers, snap peas
- Soy sauce, ginger, sesame oil for seasoning

Instructions:

1. Stir-fry chickpeas and mixed vegetables with soy sauce, ginger, and sesame oil.
2. Serve over brown rice or quinoa.

Nutritional Information:

- Calories: 300-400 per serving
- Protein: 15-20g
- Carbohydrates: 40-50g
- Fat: 10-15g

24. Turkey and Sweet Potato Hash:

Ingredients:

- Ground turkey, sweet potatoes, bell peppers
- Onion, garlic, paprika for flavor

Instructions:

1. Sauté ground turkey, sweet potatoes, and bell peppers with onion, garlic, and paprika.
2. Cook until everything is golden brown and cooked through.

Nutritional Information:

- Calories: 350-450 per serving
- Protein: 25-30g
- Carbohydrates: 30-40g
- Fat: 15-20g

25. Greek Chicken Salad Wraps:

Ingredients:

- Grilled chicken, cucumber, cherry tomatoes, feta
- Whole-grain wraps, tzatziki sauce

Instructions:

1. Mix grilled chicken, cucumber, cherry tomatoes, and feta.
2. Fill whole-grain wraps and drizzle with tzatziki sauce.

Nutritional Information:

- Calories: 300-400 per serving
- Protein: 30-35g
- Carbohydrates: 20-30g
- Fat: 10-15g

26. Broccoli and Cheese Stuffed Chicken:

Ingredients:

- Chicken breast, broccoli, cheddar cheese
- Garlic, onion powder, breadcrumbs

Instructions:

1. Butterfly chicken breast and stuff with steamed broccoli and cheddar cheese.

2. Sprinkle with garlic, onion powder, and breadcrumbs. Bake until chicken is cooked through.

Nutritional Information:

- Calories: 350-450 per serving
- Protein: 30-35g
- Carbohydrates: 10-15g
- Fat: 15-20g

27. Spinach and Mushroom Egg Muffins:

Ingredients:

- Eggs, spinach, mushrooms
- Feta cheese, salt, and pepper

Instructions:

1. Whisk eggs and fold in chopped spinach and mushrooms.
2. Pour the mixture into muffin cups, top with feta, and bake until set.

Nutritional Information:

- Calories: 200-300 per serving
- Protein: 15-20g
- Carbohydrates: 5-10g
- Fat: 15-20g

28. Teriyaki Salmon Bowl:

Ingredients:

- Grilled salmon, brown rice, broccoli
- Teriyaki sauce, sesame seeds, green onions

Instructions:

1. Place grilled salmon, brown rice, and steamed broccoli in a bowl.
2. Drizzle with teriyaki sauce and sprinkle with sesame seeds and green onions.

Nutritional Information:

- Calories: 400-500 per serving
- Protein: 30-35g
- Carbohydrates: 40-50g
- Fat: 15-20g

29. Lentil and Vegetable Soup:

Ingredients:

- Lentils, carrots, celery, onion
- Vegetable broth, garlic, cumin

Instructions:

1. Cook lentils, carrots, celery, and onion in vegetable broth with garlic and cumin.
2. Simmer until vegetables are tender.

Nutritional Information:

- Calories: 250-350 per serving

- Protein: 15-20g

- Carbohydrates: 40-50g

- Fat: 5-10g

Ingredients:

- Shrimp, corn tortillas, cabbage slaw

- Cilantro, lime, Greek yogurt for topping

Instructions:

1. Sauté shrimp with cilantro and lime.

2. Assemble tacos with corn tortillas, cabbage slaw, and a dollop of Greek yogurt.

Nutritional Information:

- Calories: 300-400 per serving

- Protein: 20-25g

- Carbohydrates: 30-40g

- Fat: 10-15g

Ingredients:

- Acorn squash, ground turkey, cooked quinoa

- Onion, garlic, sage for flavor

Instructions:

1. Roast acorn squash halves until tender.

2. Sauté ground turkey, cooked quinoa, onion, garlic, and sage. Stuff the squash halves.

Nutritional Information:

- Calories: 350-450 per serving
- Protein: 25-30g
- Carbohydrates: 30-40g
- Fat: 15-20g

32. Lemon Garlic Chicken Skewers:

Ingredients:

- Chicken breast cubes, bell peppers, red onion
- Lemon, garlic, oregano for marinade

Instructions:

1. Marinate chicken, bell peppers, and red onion in a mixture of lemon, garlic, and oregano.
2. Thread onto skewers and grill until chicken is cooked through.

Nutritional Information:

- Calories: 300-400 per serving
- Protein: 30-35g
- Carbohydrates: 5-10g
- Fat: 15-20g

33. Sweet Potato and Black Bean Quesadillas:

Ingredients:

- Whole-grain tortillas, sweet potatoes, black beans
- Cheddar cheese, cumin, paprika for flavor

Instructions:

1. Mash sweet potatoes and black beans with cumin and paprika.

2. Spread the mixture between whole-grain tortillas, add cheddar cheese, and cook until cheese is melted.

Nutritional Information:

- Calories: 350-450 per serving
- Protein: 15-20g
- Carbohydrates: 40-50g
- Fat: 15-20g

34. Mediterranean Tuna Salad:

Ingredients:

- Canned tuna, cherry tomatoes, cucumber, olives
- Feta cheese, olive oil, lemon juice for dressing

Instructions:

1. Mix canned tuna, cherry tomatoes, cucumber, and olives.
2. Drizzle with olive oil and lemon juice, then top with crumbled feta.

Nutritional Information:

- Calories: 300-400 per serving
- Protein: 25-30g
- Carbohydrates: 10-15g
- Fat: 15-20g

35. Butternut Squash and Kale Salad:

Ingredients:

- Roasted butternut squash, kale, quinoa
- Pomegranate seeds, feta, balsamic vinaigrette

Instructions:

1. Combine roasted butternut squash, kale, and quinoa.
2. Top with pomegranate seeds, feta, and drizzle with balsamic vinaigrette.

Nutritional Information:

- Calories: 300-400 per serving
- Protein: 10-15g
- Carbohydrates: 40-50g
- Fat: 10-15g

36. BBQ Chickpea and Vegetable Skewers:

Ingredients:

- Chickpeas, bell peppers, zucchini
- BBQ sauce, smoked paprika, cumin for seasoning

Instructions:

1. Toss chickpeas and vegetables in a mixture of BBQ sauce, smoked paprika, and cumin.
2. Skewer and grill until veggies are tender.

Nutritional Information:

- Calories: 250-350 per serving
- Protein: 10-15g
- Carbohydrates: 40-50g / Fat: 5-10g

37. Orange Ginger Salmon:

Ingredients:

- Salmon fillets, orange juice, ginger
- Soy sauce, honey, garlic for marinade

Instructions:

1. Marinate salmon in a mixture of orange juice, ginger, soy sauce, honey, and garlic.
2. Bake or grill until salmon is cooked through.

Nutritional Information:

- Calories: 400-500 per serving
- Protein: 30-35g
- Carbohydrates: 10-15g
- Fat: 20-25g

38. Cauliflower and Chickpea Curry:

Ingredients:

- Cauliflower, chickpeas, spinach
- Coconut milk, curry paste, turmeric

Instructions:

1. Cook cauliflower, chickpeas, and spinach in a curry sauce with coconut milk, curry paste, and turmeric.
2. Serve over brown rice.

Nutritional Information:

- Calories: 350-450 per serving
- Protein: 15-20g
- Carbohydrates: 40-50g
- Fat: 15-20g

39. Walnut and Cranberry Quinoa Salad:

Ingredients:

- Cooked quinoa, walnuts, dried cranberries
- Spinach, feta, balsamic vinaigrette

Instructions:

1. Combine quinoa, walnuts, and dried cranberries.
2. Toss with spinach, crumbled feta, and drizzle with balsamic vinaigrette.

Nutritional Information:

- Calories: 300-400 per serving
- Protein: 10-15g
- Carbohydrates: 40-50g
- Fat: 15-20g

40. Tomato Basil Chicken Zoodle Bowl:

Ingredients:

- Zucchini noodles, grilled chicken, cherry tomatoes
- Fresh basil, Parmesan cheese, olive oil

Instructions:

1. Sauté zucchini noodles with grilled chicken and cherry tomatoes.
2. Top with fresh basil, Parmesan cheese, and a drizzle of olive oil.

Nutritional Information:

- Calories: 300-400 per serving
- Protein: 30-35g
- Carbohydrates: 10-15g / Fat: 15-20g

These quick and easy recipes are designed for those hectic days when time is of the essence. By keeping the ingredients simple and the preparation minimal, these recipes ensure that even on busy days, individuals can stick to their metabolic confusion meal plan with ease.

Incorporating these sample meal plans and recipes into the metabolic confusion journey provides a practical and enjoyable approach to nutrition for endomorphs. The key lies in flexibility, variety, and a commitment to aligning dietary choices with the unique needs of endomorphic bodies.

CHAPTER SIX
THE ROLE OF EXERCISE

6.1 Importance of Exercise for Endomorphs

For individuals with an endomorphic body type, characterized by a tendency to store fat and a slower metabolism, incorporating regular exercise into their routine becomes pivotal. Understanding the importance of exercise goes beyond the pursuit of aesthetics; it becomes a fundamental aspect of managing weight, enhancing metabolic function, and promoting overall well-being.

Endomorphs often face challenges related to weight management due to their body's natural inclination to store excess calories as fat. Exercise acts as a powerful tool to counterbalance this predisposition. Regular physical activity helps in burning calories, improving insulin sensitivity, and boosting metabolism, all of which are crucial for individuals aiming to shed excess weight.

Beyond weight management, exercise plays a vital role in supporting hormonal balance, a factor that is particularly relevant for endomorphs. Hormones such as insulin, cortisol, and leptin have a direct impact on metabolism and fat storage. Engaging in consistent physical activity helps regulate these hormones, contributing to a more balanced and efficient metabolic system.

Furthermore, exercise is associated with improved mood and mental well-being. Endomorphs may sometimes struggle with feelings of frustration or disappointment in their weight loss journey. Regular exercise releases endorphins, the body's natural mood lifters, reducing stress and promoting a positive mindset.

To harness the full benefits of exercise, endomorphs should focus on a combination of aerobic exercises, strength training, and flexibility exercises. This holistic approach not only aids in weight management but also contributes to overall health and longevity.

6.2 Types of Exercises for Metabolic Confusion

Metabolic confusion, a concept centered around varying exercise routines to prevent the body from adapting to a specific regimen, holds particular significance for endomorphs. Embracing a diverse range of exercises not only enhances the effectiveness of a workout but also keeps the metabolic rate elevated, promoting continuous calorie burn.

1. **Aerobic Exercises:** Endomorphs benefit greatly from aerobic exercises, which include activities like brisk walking, running, cycling, and swimming. These exercises elevate the heart rate, promoting cardiovascular health and aiding in fat loss. The key to metabolic confusion lies in diversifying aerobic workouts, alternating between high-intensity interval training (HIIT) sessions and steady-state cardio.

   Aerobic exercises form the foundation of any well-rounded fitness routine. These activities, characterized by sustained periods of rhythmic, oxygen-dependent movement, elevate the heart rate, improving cardiovascular health and aiding in weight management. For metabolic confusion, endomorphs should alternate between different forms of aerobic exercises, such as:

   Running and Jogging: Incorporating both steady-state running and high-intensity interval running sessions provides variety and challenges the cardiovascular system.

Cycling: Whether on a stationary bike or outdoors, cycling engages the lower body muscles and offers a low-impact option for cardio.

Swimming: A full-body workout, swimming is gentle on the joints and introduces a different set of challenges, contributing to metabolic confusion.

Rowing: Rowing exercises engage various muscle groups simultaneously, providing an effective and adaptable cardio option.

2. **Strength Training:** Incorporating strength training into the exercise routine is crucial for endomorphs. While cardio burns calories during the activity, strength training builds lean muscle mass, which continues to burn calories even at rest. Compound exercises like squats, deadlifts, and bench presses engage multiple muscle groups, providing an efficient and effective workout. To implement metabolic confusion, vary the intensity, sets, and repetitions in strength training routines.

Strength training is paramount for endomorphs aiming to enhance metabolism and promote fat loss. By building lean muscle mass, individuals can elevate their basal metabolic rate, leading to increased calorie burn even at rest. Key strength training exercises include:

Compound Movements: Exercises like squats, deadlifts, bench presses, and overhead presses engage multiple muscle groups, offering an efficient way to build strength.

Bodyweight Exercises: Incorporating bodyweight exercises like push-ups, pull-ups, and planks adds variety to the routine and improves functional strength.

Resistance Training: Using resistance bands, dumbbells, or kettlebells introduces variability and challenges the muscles in different ways.

Circuit Training: Structuring workouts as circuits, where different exercises are performed consecutively with minimal rest, promotes metabolic confusion by keeping the body adaptable to changing demands.

3. **Flexibility and Mobility Exercises:** Often overlooked, flexibility and mobility exercises are vital for overall fitness and injury prevention. Endomorphs can benefit from activities like yoga or Pilates, which enhance flexibility and promote better posture. Integrating dynamic stretches and mobility drills into the routine helps keep the body agile and responsive, contributing to metabolic confusion by introducing variability.

Often overlooked, flexibility and mobility exercises play a vital role in overall fitness. These exercises improve joint range of motion, reduce the risk of injuries, and contribute to better posture. Incorporate the following into the routine:

Yoga: Yoga not only enhances flexibility but also promotes balance and relaxation, making it a valuable addition to a well-rounded routine.

Pilates: Focused on core strength, Pilates exercises contribute to overall body stability and flexibility.

Dynamic Stretching: Including dynamic stretches in the warm-up routine helps prepare the body for the workout ahead and improves overall mobility.

4. **Interval Training:** High-intensity interval training (HIIT) is a powerful tool for metabolic confusion. Alternating between short bursts of intense exercise and periods of rest or lower intensity challenges the body, preventing adaptation. HIIT workouts can include a variety of exercises such as sprints, burpees, or kettlebell swings. The unpredictability in these workouts keeps the body on its toes, fostering metabolic flexibility.

High-Intensity Interval Training (HIIT) is a powerful strategy for metabolic confusion. Alternating between short bursts of intense exercise and periods of rest or lower intensity challenges the body, preventing it from adapting to a specific routine. HIIT exercises can include:

Sprints: Incorporate short, intense sprints into the workout, whether on a treadmill, track, or outdoor space.

Burpees: A full-body exercise that combines elements of strength and cardio, burpees elevate the heart rate quickly.

Kettlebell Swings: This dynamic exercise engages the hips and lower body, providing a cardiovascular challenge while building strength.

Box Jumps: Jumping onto a box or platform requires explosive power, contributing to both cardiovascular fitness and strength.

6.3 Creating A Sustainable Exercise Routine

Creating a sustainable exercise routine is essential for endomorphs to ensure long-term success in their fitness journey. Sustainability involves finding a balance that accommodates individual preferences, lifestyle, and physical capabilities. Here are key considerations for crafting a sustainable exercise routine:

1. **Set Realistic Goals:** Begin by setting realistic and achievable fitness goals. Unrealistic expectations can lead to frustration and burnout. Whether it's losing a certain amount of weight, running a specific distance, or mastering a particular exercise, setting small, attainable goals provides a sense of accomplishment and motivation.

2. **Diversify Workouts:** To prevent boredom and maintain interest, diversify the types of exercises incorporated into the routine. This not only supports metabolic confusion but also keeps the workout engaging and enjoyable. Consider trying new activities such as dance classes, hiking, or group fitness sessions to keep things interesting.

3. **Prioritize Consistency Over Intensity:** Consistency is key when it comes to exercise. Instead of sporadic intense workouts, focus on establishing a regular routine. This approach is more sustainable in the long run and allows the body to adapt gradually, reducing the risk of injuries or burnout. Consistency builds habits, making exercise an integral part of daily life.

4. **Listen to Your Body:** Pay attention to the signals your body sends. While it's important to challenge yourself, pushing too hard without adequate rest can lead to

fatigue and injuries. Rest and recovery are integral components of a sustainable exercise routine. Incorporate rest days, prioritize sleep, and consider activities like yoga or gentle stretching on recovery days.

5. **Make it Enjoyable:** Sustainable exercise should be enjoyable. Find activities that bring joy and satisfaction. Whether it's dancing, hiking with friends, or participating in a sports league, choosing activities that align with personal preferences increases the likelihood of sticking with the routine.

6. **Adapt to Lifestyle Changes:** Life is dynamic, and routines may need adjustments based on lifestyle changes. Whether it's a busy work schedule, travel commitments, or family responsibilities, be adaptable. Find creative ways to incorporate physical activity into daily life, even during hectic periods.

The importance of exercise for endomorphs extends far beyond physical appearance. It is a key element in managing weight, improving metabolic function, and fostering overall well-being. By embracing a diverse range of exercises and creating a sustainable routine, individuals can achieve lasting health benefits and enhance their quality of life.

CHAPTER SEVEN
OVERCOMING CHALLENGES

7.1 Common Challenges for Endomorphs

Endomorphs, characterized by a tendency to store fat and a slower metabolism, often face unique challenges on their fitness journey. Understanding these challenges is the first step toward overcoming them and achieving long-term success in health and wellness.

Genetic Predisposition:

One of the primary challenges for endomorphs is their genetic predisposition to store excess calories as fat. While genetics plays a significant role in determining body type, it doesn't dictate destiny. Endomorphs may have to work harder to achieve and maintain a healthy weight, but with the right lifestyle modifications, it's entirely possible.

Metabolic Rate:

A slower metabolic rate is another common challenge. Endomorphs tend to burn calories at a slower pace, making weight management more challenging. To overcome this, it's crucial to implement strategies that boost metabolism, such as regular exercise, strength training, and a well-balanced diet.

Fat Storage Patterns:

Endomorphs often experience specific fat storage patterns, such as carrying excess weight around the midsection. This can be frustrating, as it may take longer to see visible changes. Targeted exercises and a comprehensive approach to weight loss are essential to address these specific areas.

Tendency to Plateau:

Endomorphs may find that their bodies adapt to certain exercise routines or dietary plans, leading to plateaus in weight loss. This adaptability underscores the importance of incorporating variety into workouts and regularly reassessing dietary habits.

Emotional Aspects:

The emotional aspects of weight loss can be challenging for endomorphs. Frustration, impatience, and self-doubt may arise during the journey. Building a positive mindset, setting realistic goals, and celebrating small victories are vital components of overcoming these emotional challenges.

Lifestyle Factors:

Busy lifestyles, work-related stress, and a lack of time for self-care can also impede progress. Finding sustainable ways to integrate healthy habits into daily life is essential for long-term success.

7.2 Strategies for Overcoming Plateaus

Overcoming plateaus is a common concern for individuals on a weight loss journey, especially for endomorphs. When the body becomes accustomed to a certain routine, progress may stall. Employing effective strategies can reignite progress and prevent stagnation.

Diversify Your Workout Routine:

Plateaus often occur when the body adapts to a specific exercise routine. Introducing variety is crucial. Incorporate different forms of cardio, strength training, and flexibility exercises. This not only challenges the body but also prevents boredom, making workouts more enjoyable.

Adjust Intensity and Duration:

Increasing the intensity and duration of workouts can kickstart weight loss. For cardio exercises, consider adding intervals of higher intensity. In strength training, progressively increase weights or resistance. These adjustments force the body to work harder, promoting ongoing adaptation.

Periodization:

Structured periodization involves dividing the training program into distinct phases, each with specific goals and intensities. This systematic approach prevents the body from plateauing by constantly varying the training stimulus.

Nutritional Tweaks:

Plateaus can also be related to dietary habits. Analyze your nutrition plan and adjust as needed. Ensure you're consuming a well-balanced diet with an appropriate calorie deficit for weight loss. Consider consulting a nutritionist for personalized guidance.

Hydration and Sleep:

Adequate hydration and quality sleep are often overlooked factors in weight loss plateaus. Dehydration can hinder metabolic function, while inadequate sleep disrupts hormonal balance. Prioritize both hydration and sleep for overall well-being and improved weight loss results.

Monitor Stress Levels:

High stress levels can contribute to weight loss plateaus. Stress hormones, such as cortisol, may impact metabolism. Incorporate stress-reducing activities such as mindfulness, meditation, or yoga into your routine to manage stress effectively.

Reassess Goals:

Sometimes, plateaus coincide with unrealistic or overly ambitious goals. Take the opportunity to reassess your goals. Set achievable short-term objectives and celebrate milestones along the way. This approach not only keeps motivation high but also ensures a realistic pace of progress.

7.3 Dealing with Setbacks and Staying Motivated

Setbacks are an inevitable part of any transformative journey, and staying motivated during challenging times is crucial for long-term success. Whether facing a weight loss plateau, emotional challenges, or unexpected obstacles, adopting effective strategies can help navigate setbacks and maintain motivation.

Acceptance and Adaptability:

The first step in overcoming setbacks is accepting that they are a natural part of the journey. Instead of viewing setbacks as failures, see them as opportunities for growth and learning. Being adaptable to changing circumstances is a key component of resilience.

Learn from Setbacks:

Every setback provides valuable insights. Reflect on the factors that contributed to the setback, whether it's a lapse in dietary habits, missed workouts, or emotional triggers. Use this information to adjust your approach and develop strategies to prevent similar setbacks in the future.

Seek Support:

During challenging times, seeking support from friends, family, or a community with similar goals can make a significant difference. Sharing experiences, receiving encouragement, and knowing that you're not alone can boost morale and motivation.

Reassess and Adjust Goals:

Setbacks may necessitate a reassessment of goals. If a particular goal seems unattainable or is contributing to stress, consider adjusting it. Break larger goals into smaller, more manageable milestones. This approach fosters a sense of achievement and maintains motivation.

Celebrate Non-Scale Victories:

While weight loss is a common goal, celebrating non-scale victories is equally important. Recognize improvements in strength, endurance, flexibility, or overall well-being. These achievements contribute to a positive mindset and reinforce the value of the journey beyond the number on the scale.

Incorporate Enjoyable Activities:

Maintaining motivation is easier when incorporating activities, you enjoy. Whether it's a favorite sport, outdoor activities, or dance class, making fitness enjoyable increases the likelihood of staying committed in the long run.

Visualize Success:

Visualization is a powerful tool for staying motivated. Envision your success, picture yourself achieving your goals, and focus on the positive feelings associated with reaching milestones. This mental imagery can reinforce motivation and resilience.

Practice Self-Compassion:

Be kind to yourself during setbacks. Avoid self-blame or harsh criticism. Instead, practice self-compassion by acknowledging that everyone faces challenges. Treat yourself with the same understanding and encouragement you would offer a friend in a similar situation.

Create a Supportive Environment:

Surround yourself with a supportive environment that encourages healthy habits. This includes having nutritious foods readily available, scheduling regular workout times, and minimizing triggers that may lead to setbacks.

Celebrate Progress, Not Perfection:

Striving for perfection can set unrealistic expectations. Celebrate progress, no matter how small. Recognize that the journey is a series of steps, and each step forward is a success.

Overcoming challenges, navigating plateaus, and staying motivated are integral aspects of the transformative journey for endomorphs. By embracing adaptability, seeking support, and celebrating both victories and setbacks as part of the learning process, individuals can cultivate resilience and maintain the motivation needed to achieve lasting health and wellness.

CHAPTER EIGHT
MONITORING PROGRESS AND ADJUSTING THE PLAN

8.1 Tracking Your Journey

Tracking progress is a fundamental aspect of any transformative journey, especially when embarking on a metabolic confusion meal plan designed for endomorphs. Regular monitoring allows individuals to assess the effectiveness of their efforts, identify patterns, and make informed adjustments for sustained success.

The Importance of Tracking:

Tracking encompasses various elements, including dietary habits, exercise routines, and overall well-being. It provides tangible data that goes beyond the number on the scale, offering insights into the broader aspects of health and fitness. Tracking progress is not solely about weight loss; it's about understanding how lifestyle choices impact the body and adjusting accordingly.

Methods of tracking:

Food Journaling:

Keeping a detailed food journal is a powerful tool for tracking dietary habits. Record meals, snacks, portion sizes, and hydration. This not only aids in maintaining accountability but also helps identify patterns related to energy levels, mood, and digestion.

Physical Measurements:

In addition to weight, tracking physical measurements such as waist circumference, hip circumference, and body fat percentage provides a more comprehensive view of progress. Sometimes, the scale may not reflect changes in body composition, making measurements a valuable metric.

Fitness Logs:

Documenting workouts in a fitness log allows individuals to monitor exercise consistency, intensity, and progression. Note the types of exercises, duration, and any variations in the routine. This information aids in assessing the effectiveness of the workout plan and identifying opportunities for diversification.

Emotional and Mental Well-being:

Consider tracking emotional and mental well-being as well. Note stress levels, mood, and sleep quality. These factors play a significant role in overall health and can impact the success of a metabolic confusion meal plan. Identifying correlations between emotional well-being and lifestyle choices facilitates a holistic approach to health.

Frequency of Tracking:

The frequency of tracking varies based on individual preferences and goals. Some may find daily tracking beneficial, while others may prefer a weekly or monthly approach. Consistency is key; choose a tracking frequency that aligns with your lifestyle and allows for meaningful insights.

Using Technology:

Technology offers convenient tools for tracking progress. Mobile apps and wearables can streamline the process, providing real-time data on nutrition, physical activity, and sleep. These tools often come with features for goal setting, reminders, and visual representations of progress, enhancing the overall tracking experience.

Interpreting Trends and Patterns:

As data accumulates, take time to analyze trends and patterns. Look for correlations between dietary choices, exercise routines, and changes in measurements. For example, if energy levels consistently dip after certain meals, it may indicate a need for adjustments in nutrient intake or meal timing.

Adjusting the Plan Based on Tracking:

Tracking progress is not just about observation; it's a dynamic process that informs ongoing adjustments to the metabolic confusion meal plan. If weight loss stalls, energy levels fluctuate, or emotional well-being is affected, consider the following strategies for refining the plan.

8.2 When and How to Adjust Your Meal Plan

Identifying Plateaus:

Plateaus, where weight loss or other health goals stall, are common in any fitness journey. Recognizing plateaus involves a careful analysis of progress data. If weight has remained unchanged for several weeks despite adherence to the meal plan, it may be time to consider adjustments.

Meal Plan adjustments:

Caloric Intake:

Evaluate caloric intake. If weight loss has plateaued, reassess whether the current caloric deficit is still appropriate. Metabolism can adapt to reduced calorie intake over time, necessitating periodic adjustments. Gradually reduce caloric intake or introduce occasional higher-calorie days to prevent metabolic adaptation.

Macronutrient Ratios:

The balance of macronutrients—proteins, carbohydrates, and fats—plays a crucial role in metabolic confusion. Consider adjusting macronutrient ratios to promote satiety, energy, and metabolic flexibility. Experiment with slight variations in the distribution of these nutrients while maintaining overall calorie goals.

Meal Timing and Frequency:

Experimenting with meal timing and frequency is another avenue for adjustment. Intermittent fasting, for example, can introduce variability in meal timing, potentially enhancing metabolic flexibility. Evaluate how the body responds to different meal schedules and frequencies.

Incorporate Nutrient-Dense Foods:

Emphasize nutrient-dense foods to ensure the body receives essential vitamins and minerals. Opt for a variety of colorful fruits and vegetables, lean proteins, whole grains, and healthy fats. Nutrient-dense foods contribute to overall health and well-being while supporting weight loss.

Hydration:

Adequate hydration is often overlooked but plays a significant role in metabolism. Ensure proper water intake, as dehydration can impact metabolic function. Consider incorporating herbal teas or infused water for added variety.

Listening to Your Body:

While data and tracking are valuable tools, listening to your body is equally important. Pay attention to hunger and fullness cues, energy levels, and how different foods make you feel. Adjust the meal plan based on intuitive feedback and be open to fine-tuning as needed.

Professional Guidance:

Seeking professional guidance from a nutritionist or dietitian can provide personalized insights. A professional can analyze tracking data, assess individual needs, and create a tailored plan that addresses specific challenges and goals.

8.3 Celebrating Achievements

Celebrating achievements, no matter how small, is a vital component of a transformative journey. Acknowledging progress reinforces motivation, enhances self-esteem, and fosters a positive mindset. Recognizing achievements goes beyond scale victories and encompasses various aspects of health and well-being.

Types of achievements to celebrate:

Physical Transformations:

Celebrate physical transformations, such as weight loss, changes in body measurements, or improvements in muscle tone. These achievements are tangible indicators of progress and dedication.

Fitness Milestones:

Acknowledge improvements in fitness levels and endurance. Whether it's completing a challenging workout, achieving a personal best in strength training, or mastering a new exercise, these milestones reflect increased strength and resilience.

Consistent Habits:

Celebrate the establishment of consistent and healthy habits. Whether it's adhering to a regular workout routine, prioritizing nutrient-dense foods, or staying hydrated, the consistency of positive habits is a significant achievement.

Improved Energy Levels:

Notice and celebrate improvements in energy levels and overall vitality. Feeling more energized throughout the day is a testament to the positive impact of lifestyle changes on metabolic function.

Enhanced Mood and Well-being:

Recognize improvements in mood and emotional well-being. Positive changes in mental health, reduced stress levels, and an overall sense of well-being contribute to the holistic success of the transformative journey.

Celebration strategies:

Set Milestone Goals:

Break down long-term goals into smaller, achievable milestones. Celebrate each milestone with a sense of accomplishment. These smaller victories contribute to the overall success of the journey.

Reward Yourself:

Consider implementing a reward system for reaching specific goals. Rewards can be non-food-related, such as treating yourself to a spa day, purchasing new workout gear, or enjoying a leisure activity you love.

Share Achievements:

Share achievements with friends, family, or a supportive community. Vocalizing successes not only reinforces positive behavior but also invites encouragement and celebration from others.

Create an Achievement Journal:

Maintain an achievement journal to document successes, big or small. Reflecting on achievements during challenging times serves as a reminder of progress and resilience.

Reflect on the Journey:

Take moments to reflect on the overall journey. Consider where you started, the challenges overcome, and the growth experienced. Reflecting on the transformative process enhances gratitude and motivation.

The Role of Positive Reinforcement:

Celebrating achievements serves as positive reinforcement, creating a cycle of motivation and success. Positive reinforcement strengthens the commitment to the metabolic confusion meal plan and encourages the continuation of healthy habits.

Balancing Celebrations and Goals:

While celebrations are essential, it's crucial to strike a balance between acknowledging achievements and staying focused on ongoing goals. Celebrations should complement the journey rather than derail progress. Consider incorporating moderation and mindfulness into celebratory activities.

Building a Supportive Environment:

Creating a supportive environment that acknowledges and celebrates achievements contributes to a positive mindset. Surround yourself with individuals who understand and appreciate the efforts invested in the transformative journey.

Embracing Non-Scale Victories:

Recognizing and celebrating non-scale victories is paramount. Shift the focus from solely relying on the scale to acknowledging improvements in overall health, fitness, and well-being. Non-scale victories provide a more holistic perspective on success. Monitoring progress and adjusting the meal plan is a dynamic process that requires attentiveness, adaptability, and celebration. Whether tracking dietary habits, adjusting macronutrient ratios, or celebrating achievements, these strategies contribute to the overall success of the metabolic confusion meal plan for endomorphs. By embracing a comprehensive approach to progress tracking and adjustments, individuals can navigate challenges, celebrate achievements, and achieve sustainable health and wellness.

CHAPTER NINE
REAL-LIFE SUCCESS STORIES

9.1 Inspirational Narratives

Real-life success stories are powerful motivators, offering a glimpse into the transformative journeys of individuals who have navigated challenges, embraced change, and achieved their health and wellness goals. These inspirational narratives showcase the diverse paths people have taken, demonstrating that success is attainable with dedication, resilience, and the right mindset.

Story 1: Sarah's Metabolic Transformation

Sarah, a 32-year-old endomorph, embarked on her metabolic confusion journey with a determination to reclaim control over her health. Struggling with weight management and facing the challenges associated with her body type, Sarah sought a holistic approach to transform her lifestyle.

Beginning the Journey:

Sarah started by understanding her body type and metabolism. Acknowledging the characteristics of an endomorph, she embraced the idea of metabolic confusion as a key to unlocking her body's potential. Armed with knowledge, she crafted a personalized meal plan that incorporated the principles of variety, nutrient density, and strategic meal timing.

Challenges Faced:

Sarah encountered challenges along the way, from breaking habitual eating patterns to overcoming the emotional aspects of her journey. She emphasized the importance of resilience, noting that setbacks are a natural part of the process. Instead of viewing them as failures, Sarah treated them as opportunities to learn and adapt.

Incorporating Exercise:

Recognizing the role of exercise in metabolic confusion, Sarah tailored a workout routine that combined strength training, cardiovascular exercises, and flexibility workouts. She found joy in discovering different forms of physical activity, from high-intensity interval training to yoga, ensuring a well-rounded approach to fitness.

Meal Plan Adjustments:

As Sarah progressed, she learned the art of adjusting her meal plan based on her body's response. Monitoring her progress closely, she made nuanced changes to caloric intake, experimented with macronutrient ratios, and occasionally introduced higher-calorie days to prevent metabolic adaptation.

Celebrating Achievements:

Sarah's journey was punctuated by celebrations of achievements, both small and significant. Non-scale victories became a source of motivation, from improved energy levels to enhanced mood. Sarah created a supportive environment by sharing her successes with friends and family, fostering a sense of community around her transformative journey.

Key Takeaways from Sarah's Story:

Knowledge Empowers Transformation: Sarah's story emphasizes the transformative power of understanding one's body type and metabolism. Armed with knowledge, individuals can make informed choices that align with their unique needs.

Resilience Navigates Setbacks: Sarah's journey underscores the importance of resilience in the face of challenges. Setbacks are not roadblocks but opportunities for growth. By cultivating resilience, individuals can navigate obstacles and stay committed to their goals.

Variety Enhances Enjoyment: Sarah found joy in incorporating variety into her meal plan and workout routine. This not only prevented monotony but also made the journey enjoyable. Embracing variety enhances sustainability and adherence to a healthy lifestyle.

Story 2: Mark's Metabolic Mastery

Mark, a 45-year-old endomorph, discovered the transformative potential of metabolic confusion and embarked on a journey to master his metabolism. Battling the sedentary effects of a desk job and facing metabolic challenges, Mark sought a comprehensive approach to regain vitality and reshape his physique.

Initial Challenges:

Mark's sedentary lifestyle and slow metabolism posed initial challenges. Long hours at the desk and irregular eating patterns had taken a toll on his energy levels and overall well-being. Recognizing the need for a change, Mark delved into the principles of metabolic confusion to kickstart his journey.

Tailoring Nutrition for Metabolic Flexibility:

Understanding the nutritional needs of endomorphs, Mark crafted a meal plan that prioritized macronutrient balance and nutrient density. He experimented with different meal timing strategies, introducing intermittent fasting to enhance metabolic flexibility. Mark stressed the importance of patience, noting that results take time but are worth the effort.

Strategic Workout Routine:

Mark incorporated a tailored workout routine into his daily schedule. Recognizing the significance of both strength training and cardiovascular exercises, he diversified his workouts to keep his body guessing. Mark's 28-day meal plan was complemented by exercises designed to activate his metabolism, burn fat, and improve overall fitness.

Meal Timing Strategies:

A key aspect of Mark's success was the strategic timing of meals. He experimented with meal frequency and discovered a rhythm that worked for him. Balancing weekday meals with weekend specials allowed him to enjoy his favorite foods while maintaining overall nutritional goals.

Balancing Macronutrient Ratios:

Mark paid attention to macronutrient ratios, adjusting them based on his body's response. He found a balance that supported his energy needs, muscle building, and weight management. Mark emphasized the importance of understanding individual responses to different ratios and making adjustments accordingly.

Weekend Specials and Celebrations:

Mark's approach to weekend specials was a reflection of balance. While enjoying special meals, he maintained awareness of portion sizes and overall nutritional content. Weekends became opportunities to savor food without compromising the progress he had achieved during the week.

Key Takeaways from Mark's Story:

Strategic Meal Timing is Crucial: Mark's success highlights the importance of strategic meal timing in metabolic mastery. Experimenting with meal frequency and timing can enhance metabolic flexibility and contribute to overall well-being.

Balanced Nutrition Drives Results: Mark's focus on macronutrient balance and nutrient density underscores the role of nutrition in achieving transformative results. Understanding the importance of each nutrient and balancing their intake supports overall health and fitness.

Enjoyment Sustains Commitment: Mark's incorporation of weekend specials and celebrations reflects the significance of enjoyment in sustaining long-term commitment. Balancing indulgence with nutritional awareness fosters a positive relationship with food and promotes adherence to a healthy lifestyle.

9.2 Lessons Learned from Others

In exploring real-life success stories, valuable lessons emerge that can guide individuals on their own metabolic confusion journey. These lessons offer insights into the principles, mindset, and strategies that contribute to successful transformations, providing a roadmap for others seeking similar achievements.

Lesson 1: Individualized Approaches Yield Results

One common thread among success stories is the recognition that one size does not fit all. Sarah and Mark's journeys emphasize the importance of tailoring approaches to individual needs. Understanding one's body type, metabolism, and preferences allows for the creation of a personalized meal plan and workout routine. This individualized approach not only enhances effectiveness but also promotes sustainability, as it aligns with the unique requirements of each person's body.

Lesson 2: Resilience is the Cornerstone of Success

Both Sarah and Mark faced challenges along their journeys, emphasizing the pivotal role of resilience in achieving lasting results. Setbacks, plateaus, and emotional hurdles are inevitable, but viewing them as opportunities for growth rather than insurmountable obstacles is key. Resilience empowers individuals to stay committed, learn from experiences, and navigate the complexities of their transformative journey with determination and grace.

Lesson 3: Enjoyment Fuels Adherence

The incorporation of variety, strategic meal timing, and weekend specials in these success stories highlights the significance of enjoyment in sustaining adherence. A meal plan and workout routine that individuals genuinely enjoy are more likely to become integral parts of their lifestyle. Balancing nutrition with occasional indulgences and choosing exercises that bring joy contribute to a positive relationship with health and wellness. When the journey is enjoyable, individuals are more likely to stay committed in the long run.

Lesson 4: Patience is a Virtue

Both Sarah and Mark underscore the importance of patience in the transformative process. Realizing that results take time and that the journey is a gradual progression is essential for maintaining motivation. Patience allows individuals to celebrate small victories, acknowledge progress, and stay focused on long-term goals. Understanding that transformation is a journey, not a destination, fosters a mindset that supports sustainable change.

Lesson 5: Monitoring and Adaptation are Continuous Processes

Tracking progress, adjusting meal plans, and reassessing goals are ongoing processes in successful transformations. Sarah's nuanced adjustments to her meal plan and Mark's experimentation with meal timing exemplify the dynamic nature of the journey. Regular monitoring allows individuals to identify patterns, make informed adaptations, and respond to the evolving needs of their bodies. Embracing adaptability as a constant in the transformative process is crucial for continued success.

Lesson 6: Celebrating Non-Scale Victories is Essential

Recognizing achievements beyond the scale is a central theme in both stories. Non-scale victories, such as improved energy levels, enhanced mood, and consistent habits, contribute significantly to overall well-being. Celebrating these victories fosters a positive mindset, reinforcing the value of the journey beyond numerical metrics. Embracing a holistic view of success enhances motivation and encourages individuals to appreciate the multifaceted benefits of their transformative efforts.

Lesson 7: Building a Supportive Environment Enhances Success

The importance of a supportive environment is evident in both narratives. Sharing successes with friends, family, or a community creates a network of encouragement and understanding. This support system provides motivation, empathy during setbacks, and a sense of camaraderie. Building a community that aligns with health and wellness goals reinforces commitment and contributes to the overall success of the transformative journey.

Real-life success stories offer a tapestry of inspiration, lessons, and insights for those navigating the metabolic confusion meal plan for endomorphs. From the individualized approaches of Sarah and Mark to the resilience, enjoyment, patience, and continuous adaptation woven into their journeys, these stories serve as beacons of guidance for others seeking transformation. By incorporating the lessons learned from these narratives, individuals can embark on their own unique paths to health, wellness, and metabolic mastery. The journey is not only about reaching a destination but also about embracing the transformative process with dedication, learning, and a celebration of individual successes.

CHAPTER TEN
PRACTICAL TIPS AND TOOLS

10.1 Shopping Lists for Endomorphs

Creating a well-thought-out shopping list is a foundational step in the success of a metabolic confusion meal plan tailored for endomorphs. A carefully curated list not only streamlines the shopping process but also ensures that the pantry is stocked with the right ingredients to support nutritional needs and goals. Here are practical tips for developing an effective shopping list:

Understanding Nutritional Needs:

Before crafting a shopping list, it's essential to understand the nutritional needs of endomorphs. Focus on nutrient-dense foods that provide essential vitamins, minerals, and macronutrients. Prioritize lean proteins, whole grains, fruits, vegetables, and healthy fats. This forms the basis of a well-rounded and supportive meal plan.

Variety is Key:

Incorporate a diverse range of foods to ensure a variety of nutrients. Different colored fruits and vegetables, various protein sources, and a mix of whole grains contribute not only to nutritional balance but also to the enjoyment of meals. Variety prevents monotony and enhances the overall dining experience.

Seasonal and Local Produce:

Consider including seasonal and local produce in the shopping list. Seasonal fruits and vegetables are often fresher, more flavorful, and cost-effective. Supporting local farmers also contributes to sustainable and environmentally conscious choices.

Protein Sources:

Select lean protein sources such as chicken, turkey, fish, tofu, legumes, and low-fat dairy products. These proteins are essential for muscle maintenance, metabolic support, and overall satiety. Including a mix of animal and plant-based proteins provides flexibility and caters to individual preferences.

Healthy Fats:

Incorporate sources of healthy fats, such as avocados, nuts, seeds, and olive oil. These fats contribute to satiety, support nutrient absorption, and are crucial for overall well-being. Balance is key, so include a variety of sources while being mindful of portion sizes.

Whole Grains and Fiber:

Opt for whole grains like quinoa, brown rice, oats, and whole wheat products. These grains provide fiber, which aids digestion, promotes a feeling of fullness, and supports steady energy levels. Fiber-rich foods are essential for endomorphs aiming for weight management and hormonal balance.

Dairy and Alternatives:

Include dairy or dairy alternatives rich in calcium and vitamin D. These nutrients are vital for bone health. Options like Greek yogurt, almond milk, or fortified plant-based alternatives offer choices for those with specific dietary preferences or restrictions.

Condiments and Flavor Enhancers:

Choose condiments and flavor enhancers wisely to add taste without compromising nutritional goals. Herbs, spices, low-sodium sauces, and vinegars can elevate the flavor of meals without excessive calories or additives. Be mindful of sugar and sodium content when selecting condiments.

Smart Snacking Options:

Plan for smart snacking by including options like fresh fruits, nuts, yogurt, or cut vegetables. Having healthy snacks readily available reduces the temptation to reach for less nutritious options. Pre-portioned snacks can also support mindful eating.

Meal Plan Alignment:

Align the shopping list with the pre-planned meals for the week. This ensures that all necessary ingredients are on hand, minimizing the likelihood of deviating from the meal plan. Having a clear outline of meals and snacks aids in efficient and purposeful shopping.

Flexibility for Indulgences:

While focusing on nutritious choices, allow flexibility for occasional indulgences. Including a small treat or favorite snack in moderation can contribute to a positive relationship with food and prevent feelings of deprivation.

An effective shopping list for endomorphs is built on a foundation of nutrient-dense foods, variety, and a balance of macronutrients. Tailoring the list to individual preferences, dietary restrictions, and seasonal availability enhances its practicality and ensures a well-rounded approach to nutrition.

10.2 Meal Prep Hacks

Efficient meal preparation is a cornerstone of success for those following a metabolic confusion meal plan. Meal prep not only saves time during busy weekdays but also promotes consistency in adhering to nutritional goals. Here are practical meal prep hacks for endomorphs:

Batch Cooking Basics:

Embrace batch cooking as a time-saving strategy. Prepare larger quantities of staple items such as proteins, grains, and vegetables during the weekend. These can serve as building blocks for various meals throughout the week. Portion and store them for quick assembly when needed.

Versatile Protein Options:

Cook proteins in versatile ways to accommodate diverse meals. Grilled chicken, baked fish, or roasted tofu can be used in salads, wraps, stir-fries, and more. Pre-cooked proteins expedite meal preparation while providing flexibility in creating a variety of dishes.

Pre-cut and Washed Vegetables:

Invest time in washing, cutting, and prepping vegetables in advance. Store them in portioned containers for easy access during the week. Pre-cut veggies streamline the cooking process and encourage the inclusion of more vegetables in daily meals.

One-Pan Meals:

Explore one-pan meal recipes that combine proteins, vegetables, and grains on a single baking sheet or in a skillet. These meals not only minimize cleanup but also offer a balanced combination of nutrients. Experiment with different seasoning options to add variety.

Freeze Portions for Later:

Prepare extra portions of meals and freeze them for future use. This is especially useful for those days when time is limited or unexpected events disrupt regular meal prep routines. Label and date frozen portions to keep track of freshness.

Mason Jar Salads:

Assemble salads in mason jars to maintain freshness and prevent sogginess. Start with dressing at the bottom, followed by sturdier ingredients like proteins and grains, and end with leafy greens. When ready to eat, shake the jar to distribute the dressing evenly.

Overnight Oats for Breakfast:

Simplify breakfast by preparing overnight oats. Combine oats with milk or a dairy alternative, add fruits, nuts, and seeds, and let the mixture sit in the refrigerator overnight. In the morning, a nutritious and ready-to-eat breakfast is waiting.

Portion Control Containers:

Invest in portion control containers to streamline the process of measuring and packing meals. These containers help maintain proper portion sizes, supporting both nutritional goals and weight management. Prepare meals directly into these containers for added convenience.

Theme Nights for Variety:

Designate theme nights for meal prep to add variety to the week. For example, have a "Mexican night" where you prepare meals like chicken fajitas, black bean bowls, or taco salads. This adds excitement to the meal plan and reduces decision fatigue when choosing recipes.

Pre-portioned Snack Packs:

Create pre-portioned snack packs containing nuts, seeds, or dried fruits. Having these packs readily available makes it easy to grab a healthy snack instead of reaching for less nutritious options. This promotes mindful eating and supports overall nutritional goals.

Invest in Time-Saving Appliances:

Consider investing in time-saving kitchen appliances like a slow cooker, Instant Pot, or air fryer. These appliances can significantly reduce cooking time while allowing for the preparation of flavorful and nutritious meals. Experiment with different cooking methods to find what works best for your schedule and preferences.

Labeling and Organization:

Maintain an organized refrigerator and pantry by labeling containers and organizing ingredients by category. This minimizes the time spent searching for specific items and ensures that perishable items are used before expiration.

Incorporate Family or Roommate Participation:

If applicable, involve family members or roommates in meal prep. Assigning tasks to different individuals can make the process more efficient and enjoyable. It also fosters a sense of shared responsibility for maintaining a healthy and organized kitchen.

Incorporating these meal prep hacks into the routine not only saves time but also contributes to the success of the metabolic confusion meal plan. Consistent and efficient meal preparation establishes a foundation for maintaining a healthy and balanced diet, supporting the overall well-

being of individuals, especially those with endomorphic
body types.

10.3 Time-Saving Strategies

Time-saving strategies are essential for individuals with busy schedules and incorporating them into the metabolic confusion meal plan ensures that nutrition remains a priority even during hectic days. Here are practical time-saving strategies tailored for endomorphs:

Weekly Meal Planning:

Devote time each week to plan meals for the upcoming days. Having a clear outline of what to prepare reduces decision fatigue and minimizes the likelihood of opting for less nutritious options. Designate specific days for different types of meals to add variety.

Cook Once, Eat Twice:

Adopt the "cook once, eat twice" approach. Prepare larger quantities of a particular dish and repurpose it for subsequent meals. For example, grilled chicken from dinner can be incorporated into a salad for lunch the next day. This strategy maximizes efficiency while maintaining a diverse menu.

Strategic Grocery Shopping:

Plan grocery shopping strategically to save time and avoid unnecessary trips. Create a detailed shopping list based on the weekly meal plan, and organize it according to the store's layout. This minimizes the time spent wandering through aisles and ensures all necessary items are purchased in one go.

Pre-cut and Frozen Vegetables:

Take advantage of pre-cut and frozen vegetables to expedite meal preparation. While fresh produce is ideal, pre-cut options can be a time-saving alternative. Frozen vegetables are convenient and retain their nutritional value, making them a valuable resource for quick and easy meals.

Utilize Convenience Foods Wisely:

Incorporate healthy convenience foods judiciously. While whole, minimally processed foods are ideal, certain pre-packaged items can be time-savers. For example, pre-cooked quinoa, canned beans, or pre-washed salad greens can significantly reduce prep time.

Set Up a Meal Prep Day:

Allocate a specific day each week for dedicated meal prep. Use this day to cook and portion meals, wash and cut vegetables, and organize snacks. Having prepared components readily available throughout the week streamlines daily meal assembly.

Smart Cooking Techniques:

Opt for cooking techniques that require less active time. Slow cookers, Instant Pots, and sheet pan recipes allow for hands-off cooking while delivering flavorful and nutritious meals. Experiment with different techniques to find what aligns with time constraints and preferences.

Technology-Assisted Planning:

Use technology to streamline meal planning and grocery shopping. Meal planning apps, recipe websites, and grocery delivery services can simplify the process, allowing for efficient planning and organization without the need for extensive manual effort.

Pre-portioned Ingredients:

Pre-portion ingredients whenever possible. This includes measuring out spices, condiments, and other components in advance. Having ingredients ready in the right proportions not only saves time during cooking but also ensures accurate portion control.

Delegate and Share Responsibilities:

If living with others, consider delegating or sharing meal prep responsibilities. Divide tasks based on individual preferences and skills. This not only lightens the load but also fosters a collaborative approach to maintaining a healthy kitchen.

Mindful Time Management:

Practice mindful time management to prioritize nutrition within a busy schedule. Allocate specific time slots for meal preparation and consumption. Setting aside dedicated time for meals reduces the likelihood of skipping them or resorting to less nutritious options in a hurry.

Quick and Nutrient-Dense Snacks:

Keep quick and nutrient-dense snacks readily available. This ensures that even in time-sensitive situations, individuals have access to healthy options. Options like Greek yogurt, nuts, or pre-cut fruits require minimal preparation and offer valuable nutritional benefits.

Incorporating these time-saving strategies into the routine empowers individuals to maintain a metabolic confusion meal plan effectively, even when faced with time constraints. The key is to strike a balance between efficiency and nutritional priorities, ensuring that health remains a consistent focus during a busy lifestyle.

CHAPTER ELEVEN
INTERACTIVE ELEMENTS

11.1 Self-Assessment Quiz

In the journey toward metabolic confusion mastery and a tailored meal plan for endomorphs, self-awareness is a powerful tool. A self-assessment quiz serves as an interactive element to guide individuals in understanding their unique needs, challenges, and preferences. Here's how to design and leverage a self-assessment quiz effectively:

Understanding Individual Characteristics:

Begin the self-assessment quiz by exploring endomorphic characteristics. Questions can delve into body composition, response to different types of exercises, and metabolic tendencies. Understprovidehese individual traits provides a foundation for tailoring the metabolic confusion meal plan to specific needs.

Exploring Lifestyle Factors:

Incorporate questions about lifestyle factors that impact health and wellness. This may include sleep patterns, stress levels, daily activity levels, and dietary habits. By assessing these elements, individuals gain insights into potential areas for improvement and optimization.

Identifying Dietary Preferences:

Include questions related to dietary preferences and restrictions. Understanding whether individuals have specific dietary choices, allergies, or ethical considerations ensures that the meal plan aligns with their values and is realistic for long-term adherence.

Assessing Current Physical Activity:

Explore current physical activity levels and preferences. This can involve questions about the types of exercises individuals enjoy, the frequency of workouts, and any existing fitness routines. This information guides the integration of a tailored workout routine into the metabolic confusion plan.

Evaluating Emotional and Mental Well-being:

Recognize the role of emotional and mental well-being in overall health. Questions about stress management practices, coping mechanisms, and emotional eating tendencies provide a holistic view of an individual's relationship with food and the potential impact on their journey.

Scoring and Interpretation:

Design a scoring system that allows individuals to quantify their responses. This can be a numerical scale or a categorical system. Provide clear interpretation guidelines or personalized feedback based on the total score. This feedback helps individuals identify areas of strength and areas that may require more attention.

Actionable Insights:

Ensure that the self-assessment quiz offers actionable insights. Individuals should come away with a clear understanding of their status, potential areas for improvement, and specific actions they can take to enhance their metabolic confusion journey.

Integration with Metabolic Confusion Principles:

Align the self-assessment quiz with the principles of metabolic confusion. For example, if an individual indicates a preference for certain types of exercises, incorporate these preferences into the workout routine. If stress management is identified as a concern, integrate stress-reducing practices into the plan.

Periodic Reassessment:

Encourage individuals to revisit the self-assessment quiz periodically. As their journey progresses, priorities may shift, and areas of focus may evolve. Regular reassessment ensures that the metabolic confusion plan remains dynamic and responsive to changing needs.

Engagement and Motivation:

Make the self-assessment quiz an engaging and motivational tool. Provide positive reinforcement for strengths identified in the assessment and offer encouragement for areas that may need improvement. Framing the assessment as a tool for growth and progress fosters a positive mindset.

Interactive Platforms:

Consider using interactive platforms or apps to host the self-assessment quiz. This allows for easy scoring, immediate feedback, and the integration of multimedia elements such as videos or visuals to enhance the user experience. Interactive features can enhance engagement and make the assessment process more dynamic.

A self-assessment quiz serves as a dynamic and personalized starting point for individuals embarking on the metabolic confusion meal plan. By understanding their unique characteristics, preferences, and challenges, individuals can approach their journey with a targeted and informed mindset.

11.2 Reflection Exercises

Reflection exercises are powerful tools for deepening self-awareness, fostering mindfulness, and promoting a connection between actions and outcomes. In the context of the metabolic confusion meal plan for endomorphs, reflection exercises offer individuals the opportunity to evaluate their progress, assess their mindset, and make informed adjustments. Here's how to incorporate effective reflection exercises:

Setting the Tone:

Begin reflection exercises by setting a positive and non-judgmental tone. Emphasize that reflection is not about criticism but about gaining insights. Encourage individuals to approach the exercises with openness and a willingness to learn from their experiences.

Daily Food and Mood Journal:

Introduce a daily food and mood journal as a reflection exercise. Participants can record not only what they eat but also their emotional state before and after meals. This journal provides valuable insights into the emotional connection's individuals have with food and helps identify patterns.

Mindful Eating Practices:

Incorporate mindful eating practices as reflection exercises. Encourage individuals to savor each bite, pay attention to hunger and fullness cues, and reflect on the sensory experience of their meals. This mindfulness fosters a deeper connection with food and promotes a more conscious approach to eating.

Weekly Goal Reflection:

Implement weekly goal reflection sessions. Participants can review the goals they set for the week, assess their progress, and identify any challenges encountered. This exercise allows for a realistic evaluation of goal attainment and provides an opportunity to adjust goals for the upcoming week.

Body Positivity and Acceptance:

Integrate reflection exercises that focus on body positivity and acceptance. Encourage individuals to reflect on the positive aspects of their bodies, appreciate the progress made, and cultivate a mindset of self-love. This practice contributes to a healthy relationship with one's body.

Emotional Triggers Exploration:

Guide individuals in exploring emotional triggers related to eating habits. Reflection exercises can involve identifying situations or emotions that trigger certain eating behaviors. Understanding these triggers empowers individuals to develop healthier coping mechanisms and responses.

Gratitude Journaling:

Introduce gratitude journaling as a reflection exercise. Participants can reflect on aspects of their journey that they are grateful for, whether it's improved energy levels, positive mindset shifts, or successful adherence to the meal plan. Gratitude journaling promotes a positive outlook and reinforces positive behaviors.

Feedback Loop Integration:

Establish a feedback loop as part of reflection exercises. Encourage individuals to provide feedback on the effectiveness of the meal plan, the workout routine, and any other elements of the program. This feedback loop creates a sense of collaboration and ensures that the plan remains responsive to individual needs.

Visual Progress Tracker:

Incorporate a visual progress tracker as a reflection tool. This can include measurements, photos, or visual representations of goals achieved. Visual tracking provides a tangible representation of progress and serves as a motivating factor for individuals to continue their efforts.

Celebrating Non-Scale Victories:

Guide individuals in celebrating non-scale victories through reflection exercises. This can include acknowledging improvements in energy levels, sleep quality, mood, or overall well-being. Celebrating these victories reinforces the holistic benefits of the metabolic confusion journey beyond numerical metrics.

Reflection Prompts:

Provide reflection prompts to guide individuals through the process. These prompts can include questions such as:

What positive changes have you noticed in your energy levels this week?

How have your perceptions of food and eating evolved during the program?

In what ways have you successfully navigated challenges in your journey?

What non-scale victories are you proud of this month?

Group Reflection Sessions:

Facilitate group reflection sessions for participants to share their insights and experiences. This collaborative approach fosters a sense of community and provides additional perspectives that can be valuable for individual growth. Group discussions can also offer support and encouragement.

Mindset Shift Exploration:

Encourage individuals to explore mindset shifts through reflection exercises. This may involve reflecting on changes in self-perception, beliefs about food and exercise, and overall attitudes toward health. Understanding mindset shifts enables individuals to cultivate a positive and sustainable approach to well-being.

Integration with Goal Setting:

Integrate reflection exercises with goal setting for a comprehensive approach. Reflection informs the setting of realistic and meaningful goals, creating a continuous cycle of self-assessment, adjustment, and progress. Aligning reflection with goal setting ensures that individuals are actively engaged in their journey.

Regular Check-ins:

Establish regular check-ins for reflection exercises. Whether weekly or bi-weekly, these check-ins provide designated times for individuals to pause, reflect, and recalibrate. Regularity fosters consistency and makes reflection an integral part of the ongoing metabolic confusion journey.

Therefore, reflection exercises serve as pivotal elements in the metabolic confusion meal plan, offering individuals the tools to deepen their understanding of themselves, their habits, and their progress. By fostering mindfulness, self-awareness, and positive mindset shifts, reflection becomes a dynamic force for sustained success.

1.3 Goal Setting for Success

Goal setting is a cornerstone of success in any transformative journey, and in the context of a metabolic confusion meal plan for endomorphs, it provides individuals with a roadmap for progress. Effectively integrating goal-setting elements ensures that goals are meaningful, realistic, and aligned with the principles of metabolic confusion. Here's how to implement goal setting for success:

SMART Goals Framework:

Guide individuals in setting SMART goals—Specific, Measurable, Achievable, Relevant, and Time-bound. This framework ensures that goals are clear, quantifiable, realistic, meaningful, and bound by a specific timeframe. For example, a SMART goal could be: "Complete 30-minute workout five days a week for the next four weeks."

Long-Term and Short-Term Goals:

Encourage the establishment of both long-term and short-term goals. Long-term goals provide a vision for the overarching journey, while short-term goals create actionable steps toward that vision. Short-term goals can be stepping stones that, when achieved, contribute to the fulfillment of long-term aspirations.

Goal Prioritization:

Facilitate a process of goal prioritization. Not all goals are equal in terms of urgency or impact. Help individuals identify which goals are most critical at a given point in their journey. This prioritization ensures that efforts are concentrated on areas that will yield the most significant results.

Incorporating Behavior-Based Goals:

Shift the focus toward behavior-based goals rather than outcome-based goals. Behavior-based goals concentrate on the actions and habits that lead to desired outcomes. For instance, instead of setting a goal to lose a specific amount of weight, a behavior-based goal might be to consistently follow the meal plan and exercise routine.

Personalization and Individualization:

Recognize the importance of personalization and individualization in goal setting. Everyone's journey is unique, and goals should reflect personal values, motivations, and aspirations. This approach enhances the relevance and significance of the goals, fostering a deeper commitment.

Progressive Goal Adjustments:

Acknowledge that goals may need adjustments over time. As individuals progress in their metabolic confusion journey, their circumstances, preferences, and capabilities may evolve. Encourage regular assessments of goals and the flexibility to adjust based on changing needs.

Integration with Metabolic Confusion Principles:

Align goals with the principles of metabolic confusion. For example, if the focus is on hormonal balance, a goal may involve incorporating specific foods known for their hormonal support. If weight loss is a priority, goals could revolve around creating a caloric deficit through a combination of diet and exercise.

Visual Goal Representation:

Integrate visual representations of goals to enhance motivation. This can include creating vision boards, charts, or diagrams that visually depict the desired outcomes.

Visual representations serve as constant reminders of the end goals and contribute to maintaining focus and motivation.

Goal Accountability Partners:

Encourage individuals to share their goals with accountability partners. This could be a friend, family member, or a fellow participant in the metabolic confusion program. Accountability partners provide support, motivation, and a sense of shared responsibility for goal attainment.

Celebrate Milestones:

Celebrate both small and significant milestones along the way. Acknowledging achievements, no matter how modest, reinforces a positive mindset and motivates individuals to continue striving toward their goals. Milestone celebrations contribute to a sense of accomplishment and progress.

Reflective Goal Check-ins:

Incorporate reflective check-ins for goals. Regularly assess progress, challenges encountered, and lessons learned. Reflective check-ins provide opportunities for individuals to refine their goals based on real-time experiences, fostering continuous improvement.

Encourage Goal Iteration:

Create an environment that encourages goal iteration. As individuals achieve certain goals, they may discover new aspirations or areas for improvement. Iterative goal setting allows for ongoing refinement, ensuring that the goals remain aligned with evolving priorities.

Positive Reinforcement and Encouragement:

Provide positive reinforcement and encouragement throughout the goal-setting process. Acknowledge efforts, resilience in overcoming challenges, and commitment to the journey. Positive reinforcement fosters a supportive environment that enhances motivation and confidence.

Goal Setting as a Dynamic Process:

Emphasize that goal setting is a dynamic, ongoing process. The metabolic confusion journey involves continuous learning and adaptation. Goals should evolve in tandem with individual growth, creating a sense of progression and momentum.

Effective goal setting is a dynamic and personalized process integral to the success of the metabolic confusion meal plan for endomorphs. By guiding individuals to set meaningful, realistic, and aligned goals, the journey becomes a purposeful and transformative experience, marked by continuous progress and achievement.

CONCLUSION

12.1 Recap of Key Takeaways

As we reach the conclusion of the "Metabolic Confusion Meal Plan for Endomorph" journey, it's essential to reflect on the key takeaways that have shaped this transformative experience. This recap serves as a compass, guiding individuals through the profound insights and actionable strategies that define the metabolic confusion approach tailored for endomorphs.

Understanding Your Body Type

The journey commenced with a deep dive into understanding the endomorphic body type. Acknowledging the unique characteristics, metabolism challenges, and embracing your body type were pivotal themes. By recognizing the inherent qualities of an endomorph, individuals gained a foundation for tailoring their approach to health and wellness.

Demystifying Metabolic Confusion

Chapter 2 demystified the concept of metabolic confusion, unraveling its intricacies. From comprehending what metabolic confusion is to understanding how it works and the specific benefits for endomorphs, individuals were equipped with the knowledge to make informed choices. Metabolic confusion became not just a concept but a powerful tool in the pursuit of health and vitality.

Tailoring Nutrition for Endomorphs

Nutritional needs took center stage in Chapter 3, emphasizing the importance of crafting a diet specifically attuned to endomorphic requirements. Delving into macronutrient ratios, meal timing strategies, and understanding the unique nutritional needs of endomorphs laid the groundwork for a personalized and sustainable meal plan.

Crafting Your Metabolic Confusion Meal Plan

Building on nutritional insights, Chapter 4 guided individuals in crafting a metabolic confusion meal plan. From constructing a balanced plate to making optimal food choices and strategizing meal timing, this chapter empowered individuals to create a roadmap for nourishing their bodies in alignment with metabolic confusion principles.

Sample Meal Plans and Recipes

Practicality met variety in Chapter 5, where sample meal plans and recipes transformed theory into actionable steps. Weekday meal plans, weekend specials, and quick recipes for busy days provided a diverse and flavorful array of options, ensuring that the metabolic confusion journey was not only effective but also enjoyable.

The Role of Exercise

Exercise emerged as a vital component in Chapter 6, underscoring its importance for endomorphs. From understanding the significance of exercise to exploring different types of exercises for metabolic confusion and creating a sustainable exercise routine, this chapter laid the foundation for a holistic approach to well-being.

Overcoming Challenges

Chapter 7 addressed the inevitable challenges that arise on any transformative journey. From common challenges for endomorphs to strategies for overcoming plateaus and dealing with setbacks, individuals were equipped with resilience and tools to navigate hurdles and stay steadfast on their path.

Monitoring Progress and Adjusting the Plan

Reflecting on progress became paramount in Chapter 8, where tracking the journey, knowing when and how to adjust the meal plan, and celebrating achievements took center stage. This chapter reinforced the dynamic nature of the metabolic confusion approach, where adaptability ensures sustained progress.

Real-Life Success Stories

In Chapter 9, real-life success stories illuminated the transformative potential of the metabolic confusion meal plan. Inspirational narratives and lessons learned from others showcased the diverse pathways to success, fostering a sense of community and motivation among individuals embarking on their own journeys.

Practical Tips and Tools

Practicality and efficiency were key themes in Chapter 10, offering valuable tools such as shopping lists for endomorphs, meal prep hacks, and time-saving strategies. These insights provided the practical foundation for seamlessly integrating the metabolic confusion approach into daily life.

Interactive Elements

Chapter 11 introduced interactive elements to personalize the journey further. From self-assessment quizzes that foster self-awareness to reflection exercises promoting mindfulness and goal setting for success, these elements empowered individuals to actively engage with their unique metabolic confusion experience.

Conclusion:

Now, as we revisit these key takeaways, it's evident that the metabolic confusion meal plan for endomorphs is not just a diet; it's a holistic approach to well-being. It intertwines nutrition, exercise, mindset, and practicality, recognizing that health is a multifaceted journey.

The metabolic confusion approach acknowledges that one size does not fit all. It embraces the uniqueness of endomorphic individuals, offering a tailored strategy that aligns with their metabolism, body type, and lifestyle. Through understanding metabolic confusion, crafting personalized meal plans, incorporating exercise, and overcoming challenges, individuals have not merely adopted a diet but have embarked on a transformative lifestyle.

12.2 Encouragement for The Reader's Journey

As we conclude this transformative journey, it's essential to offer encouragement to every individual who has embarked on the metabolic confusion meal plan for endomorphs. Your commitment to understanding your body type, embracing metabolic confusion principles, and crafting a personalized approach to health is commendable.

You Are Unique:

Embrace the fact that you are unique. Your body type, metabolism, and preferences are distinct, and the metabolic confusion approach celebrates this individuality. What works for others may not work the same way for you, and that's perfectly okay. Embracing your uniqueness is a strength, not a limitation.

Progress, Not Perfection:

Recognize that the journey is about progress, not perfection. Every step you take, every healthy choice you make, and every lesson you learn contributes to your overall well-being. Celebrate the small victories and understand that setbacks are part of the journey. What matters most is your commitment to progress.

Mindset Matters:

Your mindset is a powerful force on this journey. Cultivate a positive and resilient mindset that sees challenges as opportunities for growth. Approach setbacks with a curious and learning mindset, understanding that each obstacle is a stepping stone toward greater understanding and success.

Listen to Your Body:

Your body is constantly communicating with you. Listen to its signals, whether it's hunger, fullness, fatigue, or satisfaction. Pay attention to how different foods and exercises make you feel. Your body is a wise guide on this journey, and tuning in to its cues fosters a harmonious relationship with your health.

Celebrate Your Achievements:

Take time to celebrate your achievements, both big and small. Whether it's reaching a fitness milestone, consistently following your meal plan, or experiencing improved energy levels, these achievements are markers of your dedication and progress. Celebrate them as evidence of your commitment to a healthier lifestyle.

Adaptability Is Key:

The metabolic confusion approach is not a rigid set of rules but a flexible framework that adapts to your evolving needs. Embrace adaptability as a key principle. If a particular strategy isn't yielding the expected results, be open to adjusting and refining your approach. Your journey is unique, and so is your path to success.

Community and Support:

Lean on the support of the community around you. Whether it's friends, family, or fellow individuals on a similar journey, the power of community cannot be overstated. Share your experiences, learn from others, and offer support in return. A supportive community enhances the richness of the journey.

Reflect and Reassess:

Regularly take time to reflect on your journey. Assess what is working well, identify areas for improvement, and reassess your goals. This reflective practice ensures that your approach remains aligned with your evolving aspirations and helps you stay focused on continuous improvement.

You Are More Than a Number:

Remember that you are more than a number on a scale. The metabolic confusion approach goes beyond conventional measures of success. Improved energy levels, enhanced mood, better sleep, and overall well-being are equally significant indicators of your progress. Value and celebrate the holistic benefits of your journey.

A Journey, not a Destination:

Lastly, view this as a journey, not a destination. Health and well-being are lifelong pursuits, and the metabolic confusion approach provides you with enduring principles to navigate this journey. Enjoy the process, savor the experiences, and relish the continuous growth that accompanies your commitment to a healthier lifestyle.

In concluding this transformative chapter, remember that the metabolic confusion meal plan for endomorphs is more than a book; it's a companion in your journey toward optimal health. May this journey be filled with self-discovery, empowerment, and the profound joy that comes from prioritizing your well-being. The road ahead is bright, and you have the tools to make it an extraordinary adventure.